Y0-BRM-096

# Praise for
# the HERBAL KITCHEN

"I learned a lot from *The Herbal Kitchen*, and I'm keeping it in my kitchen so I can refer to it often. I love this book!" —Christiane Northrup, MD, author of the *New York Times* bestseller *Women's Bodies, Women's Wisdom*

"*The Herbal Kitchen* contains the most extensive list of recipes using herbs you will find anywhere. Your food becomes your medicine, as it always has been, and through the gift of Kami McBride's recipes, this ancient usage of herbs remains alive." —Pam Montgomery, herbalist, educator, and author of *Plant Spirit Healing* and *Partner Earth*

"Plants have long been humanity's powerful and generous allies, providing us with daily nourishment, wellness, support, and joy. The more we commune with these botanical friends, the more they enrich our lives, and *The Herbal Kitchen* inspires us to invite them to each and every meal. If you long for food filled with nature's color, vitality, and love, this is the guide you seek." —Julie Bailey, herbalist, gardener, and co-owner of Mountain Rose Herbs

"*The Herbal Kitchen* is a treasure chest of delicious, nutritious recipes that will delight and tantalize your taste buds while they nourish and heal your body, mind, and spirit. McBride's deep connection and intricate knowledge of all things herbal shines through on every page. Both the beginner and the seasoned herbalist will find refreshing, exciting recipes and ideas in this outstanding book!" —Jane Bothwell, Dandelion Herbal Center

"Kami McBride has created an essential, comprehensive, and beautifully written book. It shows us the way to weave the practical magic of herbal remedies—cooking, gathering, making medicine—into the strands of our lives and the lives of our loved ones. Illuminated with personal anecdotes, it is easily accessible to beginners and inspiring to seasoned herbalists. *The Herbal Kitchen* is a beautiful recipe for self-empowerment and reconnection to the natural world." —Donna Chesner, Southwest School of Botanical Studies

"*The Herbal Kitchen* is written by a practicing herbalist, seasoned gardener, and medicine maker (no armchair herbalist here!). Kami has imbued this book with a sense of joy, practical knowledge, and deep wisdom, and with her guidance, you will deepen your knowledge and understanding of the many healing herbs and foods found in your kitchen." —Candis Cantin, author of *The Herbal Tarot* and *Pocket Guide to Ayurvedic Healing*

"Thank you, Kami McBride, for bringing back the value of herbs and spices in *The Herbal Kitchen*. An inspiration for both new and advanced herbalists alike, this book combines herbalism with nutrition in a user-friendly, inexpensive way. What better way to take a culinary trip around the world, play with flavor, and bring us back home to growing our own fresh herbs?" —DeAnna Batdorff, founder of the dhyana Center

"In *The Herbal Kitchen*, Kami McBride reminds us of the earth's bountiful food and medicine. With over two hundred fifty herbal recipes you'll easily have the practical knowledge and inspiration to cultivate your own herbal kitchen. Follow Kami's guidance and you'll soon be immersed in seasonal bounty and amazing your friends and family with delicious herbal drinks, smoothies, cordials, pestos, and more. —Rosalee de la Forêt, author of *Alchemy of Herbs: Transform Everyday Ingredients into Foods and Remedies that Heal*

"Looking to brighten your kitchen with the medicine and flavor of herbs? *The Herbal Kitchen* is infused with grounded and practical herbal wisdom, coupled with culinary inspiration and know-how. Kami's love of botanicals shines right through the pages—you'll make quick friends with the herbs she features—and your kitchen cupboards will be forever transformed." —Juliet Blankespoor, director of the Chestnut School of Herbal Medicine

"*The Herbal Kitchen* makes using herbs effortless. It will help you fill your home with delectable herbal concoctions to share with friends and family and offer ways to enhance your well-being, support self-care, and so much more. Everyone from the newcomer to the seasoned herbalist will discover new ways of using common culinary and medicinal plants with McBride's abundant recipes." —Autumn Summers, California School of Herbal Studies, lead educator at Herb Pharm

"*The Herbal Kitchen* is a beautifully written guide to expanding your herbal repertoire. This is a book that can bring more fun, flavor, and health into your life." —Brigitte Mars, author of *Rawsome!* and *The Desktop Guide to Herbal Medicine*

"*The Herbal Kitchen* is a tremendous resource. Everything you ever wanted to know about the healing power of herbs and spices is nicely tucked within these pages. This is a must-have for everyone's kitchen." —Rebecca Katz, author of *The Cancer-Fighting Kitchen: Nourishing, Big-Flavor Recipes for Cancer Treatment and Recovery*

"Be prepared for a whole new way of thinking about herbs. Kami McBride resurrects traditional knowledge of herbs' medicinal and culinary attributes for use in the modern kitchen." —Ann Vileisis, author of *Kitchen Literacy: How We Lost Knowledge of Where Food Comes From and Why We Need to Get It Back*

"*The Herbal Kitchen* reminds me of why I dove head first into herbal medicine. McBride inspires you to take your own plunge into the joys of plant medicine and to give up shelves in your kitchen for jars of roots, leaves, and flowers. She takes you by the hand down the herbal path and shows you how easy it can be. There is always room for another herb book on the shelf and *The Herbal Kitchen* is a must." —Dr JJ Pursell, herbalist and author of *The Herbal Apothecary*

"A joyful celebration of practical, sensual herbal recipes! Kami's beautiful new book brims with delicious recipes that help budding herbalists and gardeners discover the bounty in their backyard. The recipes are simple and practical yet creative—

the unique combinations of flavors excite the senses and teach you how to better enjoy herbs and spices. Together, they indulge you in the herbal lifestyle—not just for medicine, but plants and recipes that perk up your senses and make life more pleasurable." —Maria Noël Groves, herbalist and author of *Body into Balance* and *Grow Your Own Herbal Remedies*

"Full of tasty remedies and everyday delights, *The Herbal Kitchen* provides multiple variations and ideas for each type of recipe to get your creative juices flowing! Easy, sustainable, and deliciously useful." —Holly Bellebuono, MPA, CH, herbalist and author of *The Healing Kitchen* and *An Herbalist's Guide to Formulary*

"In *The Herbal Kitchen*, Kami McBride weaves an enticing invitation to dive into the art, rich tradition, and flavor of kitchen medicine. An herbal, a recipe book, and a home remedy companion all at once, I am inspired to learn, grow, cook, and share. This plethora of incredible recipes, in-depth plant profiles, and McBride's years of experience and passion will give you all the tools you need to stock your herbal pantry with condiments and remedies for lasting health." —Brittany Wood Nickerson, herbalist, owner of Thyme Herbal, and author of *Recipes from the Herbalist's Kitchen* and *The Herbal Homestead Journal*

"*The Herbal Kitchen* is a breath of fresh air and more. It is full of simple and convenient tips to transform 'weeds and waste' into exotic and nourishing culinary delights." —Margaret Beeson, naturopathic physician

"No kitchen is complete without the treasure trove of botanical wisdom found in this wonderful book!" —Deanna Minich, PhD, CN, nutritionist and author of *Whole Detox* and *The Rainbow Diet*

# The Herbal Kitchen

Bring lasting health to you and your family
with 50 easy-to-find common herbs and over 250 recipes

## KAMI McBRIDE

FOREWORD BY

## ROSEMARY GLADSTAR

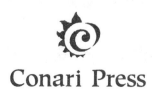

Conari Press

This edition first published in 2019 by Conari Press, an imprint of
Red Wheel/Weiser, LLC
With offices at:
65 Parker Street, Suite 7
Newburyport, MA 01950
*www.redwheelweiser.com*

Copyright © 2019 by Kami McBride
Foreword copyright © 2019 Rosemary Gladstar
All rights reserved. No part of this publication may be reproduced or transmitted in any form or
by any means, electronic or mechanical, including photocopying, recording, or by any information
storage and retrieval system, without permission in writing from Red Wheel/Weiser, LLC. Reviewers
may quote brief passages. Previously published in 2010 by Conari Press, ISBN: 978-1-57324-421-3.

ISBN: 978-1-57324-745-0
Library of Congress Cataloging-in-Publication Data available upon request.

Cover design by Kathryn Sky-Peck
Cover photograph © iStock
Interior illustrations: pages 31, 33, 34, 36, 38, 39, 41, 44, 46, 47, 50, 52, 54, 56, 60, 63, 65, 66, 68, 70, 71,
73, 78, 82, 83, 85, 86, 88, 93, 94, 97, 101, 104, 106, 108, 186 © Dover; pages 15, 29, 89, 99, 110, 113, 128,
138, 152, 168, 185, 197 ,207, 218, 231 © dreamstime.com; pages 30, 63, 91 courtesy of CLKR;
page 80 © Getty.
Author photograph © Michael Conyers

Printed in the United States of America
LB
10  9  8  7  6  5  4  3  2  1

*This book is dedicated to my mother.*
*Her never-ending love and support*
*inspired me to follow my heart.*

# Contents

# Acknowledgments

Thank you to Red Wheel Weiser and Conari Press for helping me to make this book a reality. Thank you to all my teachers who have helped guide and inspire my work and life. I am very grateful to everyone who has participated in my classes over the years; being with all of you has shaped and given an immeasurable depth to my life. Thank you to everyone who has been a part of this wonderful journey learning about plants. I am forever grateful for the beauty and mystery of plants and how they continue to be such extraordinary teachers. My wish is that these pages benefit and bring health to all.

# Preface

Thirty years ago, I made a commitment to honor the earth by resurrecting the herbal kitchen in our homes to help people practice kitchen medicine every day. I have dedicated my life to speaking, writing, and teaching people how to use plant medicines to take care of themselves and to help raise the next generation of children to do the same.

My healing journey began at nineteen years old, when I was diagnosed with a brain tumor. My surgeon had some news for me. He said, "No-one's going to tell you this, but stop the medication you're taking. It causes tumors and it's the reason why you needed this surgery." Suddenly I realized that I was a statistic—I was one of the number of people who develop a serious condition from taking prescription medication.

This shocking news stopped me in my tracks, to say the least. I started to read the information sheet that comes with medications. You know, that little white paper with microscopic writing that's been folded fifty times? If you are going to take a pill, you actually want to read that paper, so you can decide if the gamble is worth it. I also noticed that every elder in my life was taking multiple medications.

I asked myself, "Isn't there another way? A better way we can take care of ourselves?" I have since learned that our lives are very much guided by the questions we ask, and these questions set the course for me. Soon after, I heard the phrase "holistic health" for the very first time. "What is that, I thought?" And so, it began, one thing after another led me down the path to the amazing world of healing with herbs.

I felt a desire to teach what I had been learning about herbs to help people realize that there are other choices for taking care of themselves. I had a vision to gather the women to make herbal foods and medicines together as a way to honor the earth and revive the art of home herbal care. I acted on that vision and have been doing this work ever since.

I wrote *The Herbal Kitchen* to help people, to show them that using herbal medicine didn't have to be complicated. When the book was first published, there was an "Herbal Renaissance" afoot. People were getting fed up with the sea of advertisements for over-the-counter drugs and they were hungry for other ways to support their health and treat common ailments. The Herbal Renaissance is now a full-on cultural movement. People are seeking out information about medicinal plants and learning how to use them to prevent and heal illness, to ease stress and help them sleep, and more.

Today, there are hundreds of books and thousands of herbal how-to blogs—it can be overwhelming and difficult to organize or incorporate all the information. In one week, we are exposed to more information than our great-grandmothers were in years, but it's impossible to download generations of herbal knowledge with just the press of a button. No matter how information and online savvy we are, information doesn't digest without experience. The experience that makes your herbal journey real starts in the kitchen.

Most of us have an amazing apothecary just waiting to be discovered in our homes. The medicine is right there in our kitchens, we just forgot about the depth of its value. I like to think of this remembering as a warming of the hearth. The kitchen hearth is where we transform the gifts of the earth's harvest into food and medicine that keeps our family well.

Somewhere along the line this art and craft became drudgery. We subscribed to the cult of busy and we no longer had time to devote to feeding ourselves and our families. We lost the joy to be had in transforming the sunlight captured by plants into nourishment for our own cells.

Modern life has led to multiple layers of cultural disruption. The ancestral food, medicines, and stories are gone. Many of our celebrations are guided by the media and screens, defining when and what they should be. The hearth calls us back to the kitchen, where authentic experience and connection are rooted in the harvest of the earth and the turning of the seasons. We gather people around to notice nature's gifts, to celebrate and share delicious, healing food inspired by the abundance of the harvest and made with love.

I have the good fortune of seeing the children and grandchildren of many of my students who were raised with herbs and how that has impacted their lives. It is amazing to witness their confidence as they take care of their families' health in a proactive way. Many of them have created herbal programs in their schools and camps and have planted neighborhood herb gardens. They are evidence that the tide has turned: herbalism is alive and well and it is the healing balm we need for the times we're living in.

When we bring our hearts and hands back into how we build our lives and our food, our meals become our medicines. By bringing the earth into our home, we thank and honor her by creating remedies that are a source of vitality in our lives. This is the knowledge that lives deep in our bones. If you weren't raised with this teaching, you may not know it is there. But once you get a taste of it, there is no going back. You have been activated. The impulse to live closer to the earth is now moving through you. You are part of the intelligence that has awakened to move from a culture that desecrates the earth to one that is recreating a sacred covenant with all that sustains life. Welcome home to your herbal kitchen.

It is amazing how much connection and opportunity opens up when you write your soul down on paper. So much gratitude and goodness has come to me from this little book. I hope it brings the same to you.

Thank you, it is such a joy to be on this journey.
Kami McBride

# Foreword

Herbalism and herb books have become quite the hot topic these past few years, and there are herb books on any subject one could imagine exploring the broad territory that herbalism embraces. Quite the change from only a few years back, when one would want books on herbs and herbal healing and find they were far and few between. Today, quite thankfully, my library shelves are heavily stacked with books on plant spirit medicine, wild crafting and identification, herbal healing and herb lore, the latest most popular herbs, using herbs with drugs and medication and contraindications, and herbal medicine as a clinical practice. You name it, big book or small, colorfully laid out or plainly printed, each herb book holds at least a few gems and often many about this intriguing field of study that I have been impassioned with for most of my life. But few touch my heart the way Kami McBride's *The Herbal Kitchen* does. It embraces all that I love most about this ancient healing tradition and reminds me of how necessary our relationship to plants is in our world today.

In *The Herbal Kitchen* sits the rich green heart of herbalism in all its abundance, simplicity, and practicality. Medicines are made, recipes exchanged, and wise adages passed along to the reader. One can almost smell the flowers, taste the cup of tea in hand, so homespun and real are the teachings that Kami shares. She artfully guides us through garden and field ripe with earth's abundance, then leads us back into the heart of the household, the earthy abode of the kitchen. There, amidst pots and pans, herb jars, and baskets overflowing with the lush harvest of fragrant plants, all that is best about the tradition of herbal healing comes forth,

*"Herbs and spices are a gift from nature. We are nature and the plants have an affinity with our bodies . . . they are our allies."*
(from *The Herbal Kitchen*)

as Kami generously shares not only recipe and remedy, but wisdom passed down through time.

With the simplest of ingredients and always an eye for what is practical and doable, Kami guides us to create recipes for health and healing and weaves the magic and power of herbs back into our daily lives. Every recipe embraces that wise old adage, "food is our best medicine." Within the limitless range of the kitchen lies the pathway to wellness. As Kami makes obvious, "this is a book about reclaiming the art of using herbs in our daily food routines and developing a deeper understanding of our relationship between food and wellness."

*"The culture of our kitchen environment is the space we create to nurture and care for ourselves and our families...."*

But this is far more than just a book of recipes and remedies. Kami embraces all that's real and honest, traditional and practical, about the green world, and she generously, with spice and vigor, offers her warm insights for all of us to savor. It's sweetly delicious, like the elderberry syrup, Rose Delight Honey, and Benedictine liqueur, (recipes she shares along with the stories that accompany them). One can feel the grandmothers with her, guiding her, whispering their ancient wisdom and infusing it into the very teachings that Kami shares so warmly with us. Perhaps that is one of the reasons I love this book so much; it offers a sweet antidote to the sometimes stale modernism of so many herb books written today. In Kami's *The Herbal Kitchen* I am reminded of all that I love most about this ancient tradition of healing, how it's been passed down through the ages, from grandmother to granddaughter, grandfather to grandson; how it embraces simplicity and humbleness, while being grand and noble at the same time. And how

*"I keep a watchful eye for what the earth has to offer, paying my respects by nourishing my body and soul with the harvest.*
(from The Herbal Kitchen)*

it offers us the best kind of medicine, the kind that feeds the heart as well as the body, reaching deeply into the sacred places of our souls to heal us from the inside out.

Read deeply; this is a book that will nourish heart and soul, body and spirit with the rich harvest of the green world. And yes, another book to add to my shelves of green literature. This one, however, goes on the top shelf, where I house most of my favorite tomes and the ones I use most often.

Rosemary Gladstar, herbalist and author
From her mountain home in Vermont

# Introduction

Do you enjoy eating garlic bread? Does oregano always find its way into your spaghetti sauce? Do you garnish potato salad with paprika? Then you are participating in the ancient tradition of using herbs to enhance the health benefits and digestibility of your food.

Herbs in the kitchen not only augment the flavor of what we eat, they support our overall health and wellness on a daily basis. Whether you are a seasoned cook or just cutting your teeth in the kitchen, these pages assist you in nurturing and healing yourself and your loved ones.

Did you know that stuffing your turkey with sage helps keep away the colds that begin circulating around Thanksgiving? Or that adding ginger to a fish meal kills pathogens found specifically in fish? And when you sprinkle fennel into your meat marinades, it helps you digest the fat in the meat more easily. These pages discuss many herbs and spices that you already have in your kitchen. My hope is that you will be inspired to think of your spice rack as more than a source of flavor. It is also a medicine chest, full of healing remedies that can help you keep your family well.

I am so grateful that you have picked up this book. Who do you know who is entrusted with preparing food for their family or tending to the wellness of those around them? Please get a copy for them also. *The Herbal Kitchen* is about using herbs to prevent illness and elevate the nutritional value of whatever is prepared in your kitchen. This essential information can help you use herbs in your foods to more efficiently address the seasonal and specific health needs of the people for whom you prepare meals.

There is an extraordinary pharmacy waiting for you right in your own kitchen. With just a handful of herbs, you can begin to fortify the nutrient and therapeutic density of your meals. Adding valuable vitamins, minerals, and digestive aids to your food takes little effort.

Let's become more intimate with the spice cabinet. Using medicinal herbs doesn't have to be foreign and difficult or take years of college to understand. We can begin with what we have on hand and already have a relationship with. Most of the herbs in this book are common household items; you don't even have to buy anything. You just get to realize the full array of benefits of what currently sits in your cupboards. Let's take cinnamon for example; most everyone has cinnamon and has used it to liven up their oatmeal or pumpkin pie mix. Cinnamon is a highly medicinal herb with hundreds of health and kitchen medicine applications. It is a first-rate cold and flu prevention agent and remedy, and it offers relief from menstrual cramps, allergy symptoms, coughs, and much more. The same thing holds true for all the common spices: oregano, garlic, sage, cloves, and pepper all contain healing attributes that inspire good food and good health.

Food is one of our most powerful medicines. We create millions of cells every few seconds. What we eat is what we use to build those cells. Most of the kitchen herbs promote nutrient digestion and assimilation, helping to increase the quality of the cells that make up our tissue and organs. Many culinary herbs activate the circulatory system, contributing to more efficient dispersal of beneficial nutrients. Culinary herbs are also a surprisingly effective source for helping to calm the body while eating, so you can relax and enjoy the amazing process of digesting life into life. When you understand the comprehensive digestive support that the spice rack offers, you realize the value of using herbs to practice preventive health care while you eat.

Adding ginger to increase the digestibility of chicken, pacifying the mucus-forming effects of yogurt with cardamom, whipping up a fennel tea when someone complains of a stomachache—this is the creative, health-giving art of having fun with herbs in the kitchen. Who knows how long that stomachache would have persisted or who else would have contracted it were it not quelled with an herbal remedy? The small act of adding healing herbs and spices to our food is one of many things we do to nurture and care for ourselves and those around us.

Writing this book has been an alchemical distillation of more than twenty years of my personal hobby and professional occupation. Years and years of classes in herbal medicine and herbal cooking are concentrated into the chapters before you. It has been an exhilarating adventure having the opportunity of placing my botanical kitchen curriculum into your hands. I sincerely hope that you are inspired to use the accumulated experience in this book to enhance your health, save money, make your food taste better, nurture your relationship with the earth and the people around you, and to have fun.

## DISCLAIMER

This book is intended to be used as an educational tool. The suggestions described in this book are not a substitute for appropriate counseling, diagnosis, and treatment from a qualified medical professional. If you are taking medications, consult your health care practitioner before taking herbs. This book is about culinary uses of herbs and spices. If you want to take these plants in larger doses to achieve more therapeutic effects, please consult your health care practitioner.

If you are taking medications, consult your physician before taking herbs. Many herbs are contraindicated or inadvisable in chronic and acute diseases. If you have a health challenge, consult with your health care practitioner before using herbs. It is best to be cautious when using herbs and spices while pregnant. Carminative and antispasmodic herbs that are commonly found in foods can stimulate the uterus and are not recommended for use during pregnancy. Please consult with your midwife and health care practitioner before using herbs and spices during pregnancy. Never taste an herb if you are not sure what it is. Only use herbs that have been accurately identified.

PART ONE

# Your Herbal Kitchen

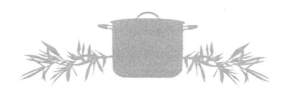

# CHAPTER 1

# Kitchen Medicine and Culinary Culture

Many people use herbs and spices in their cooking, often because these food combinations are what they grew up with, because a recipe calls for herbs and spices, or because it is just in the ether that you can't make spaghetti sauce without oregano. Awareness of the health benefits is not in the forefront of why we use spices. Often people serve food combinations without realizing the medicinal value of what they are cooking with. Whether we appreciate it or not, the use of herbs to support optimum digestion is embedded in garnishes, sauces, dressings, and condiments. It is common to serve chicken with curry sauce, garlic with eggs, and mint jelly with lamb. You will find cinnamon applesauce with pork chops, dill pickles with lunchmeat sandwiches, juniper berries with cabbage, and ginger with fish. Mustard seed would sit in my mom's cupboard all year. She didn't often use mustard seed, but she always pulled it out for the special occasion of preparing corned beef and cabbage on St. Patrick's Day. She is of Irish heritage, and that is the dish that her mother and grandmother had prepared in celebration of the holiday. It is a good thing she used the mustard seed, otherwise that corned beef would sit like a wet log in the stomach.

Herbs and spices are a gift from nature. We are nature, and plants have an affinity with our bodies. They are our allies, not only enlivening the taste of our food but also working in hundreds of ways to keep our bodies healthy. When I add thyme to spaghetti sauce, I think about how it is helping to keep my family from catching a cold or getting a stomach bug from something in the food.

We all have to eat, and we need whole, seasonal foods to be healthy. We need herbs and spices not only for flavor, but also to help us digest and assimilate what we eat. If you look through old cookbooks, you'll see that each food is paired with specific spices. Sage goes with turkey, pepper spices cheese sauces, fennel accompanies sausage, celery seed garnishes root vegetables, mustard and horseradish are served with beef, and the list goes on. As we have come to rely on packaged foods preserved with salt, sugar, and chemicals, we use fewer herbs and spices to flavor and preserve our food. This book is about reclaiming the art of using herbs in our daily food routines and developing a deeper understanding of the relationship between what we eat and our wellness.

As an herbalist, I talk to many people about health. The conversation eventually leads to questions about what to do for a sick child, friend, or family member or how to prevent them from becoming ill. Since food is one of our primary medicines, I always begin with exploring what a family eats that either invites or deters illness. What I have noticed is that today fewer women cook, and especially many younger women possess less comprehensive cooking skills than women their age fifteen years ago. It is surprising how many women begin our sessions by saying "I don't cook." The pervasiveness of convenience meals has contributed to a way of life that continually erodes our food and body knowledge base.

As more and more of our meals come neatly wrapped in neon-colored packages, the meat and vegetables are watered down with cheap oils, and the spices are replaced by chemicals. The imposter spice additives deceive our taste buds into craving fraudulent foods that are an assault to our physical strength and intelligence. Food becomes a burden to our body instead of a source of vitality. We lose our sense of taste for what nourishes a strong body. We disassociate with where our food comes from or what it takes to prepare it. I have heard children say that their food comes from a vault under the grocery store.

One of the many advantages of increasing your herb quotient in meal preparations is the vitamin and mineral content of herbs and spices. The spice cabinet and garden are abundant in mineral-rich herbs. Chemical farming practices have depleted the soil of nutrients that would normally transfer into our vegetables. The breadth of flavor in a vegetable is an indicator of its mineral content. Mineral-rich vegetables have a full, sweet taste. Vegetables devoid of minerals taste like nothing; I refer to them as cardboard vegetables. Many chronic diseases develop from nutrient deficiency. With the widespread consumption of prepackaged and conventionally farmed foods, we are experiencing the phenomenon of being overfed yet undernourished. Eat fresh, whole, organic, and locally grown food and add herbs to as many meals as possible.

I spend a significant amount of time with students and clients exploring strategies for how, when, and what to eat. This basic knowledge of nourishing ourselves is absent from so many people's lives. If you weren't raised with the appreciation of homemade, well-spiced, whole foods, it can be an overwhelming task to learn from scratch.

The recipes in this book are simple and for everyone, both seasoned healthy eaters and those who are looking to make a change for the better in their dietary habits. You can begin by choosing one or two herbs or spices to work with and make as many things as you can with them. You can also choose one medium to work with; obsessions with herb-infused oils have been known to happen. Make as many varieties of herbed oils as you can stand and then just let them have their way in your kitchen.

The herbal crafting that is abundant in my food preparation is an embodied art of asking, "How do I better understand the food and medicine that the earth provides? How do I better know and care for my body?" This book is a piece of the lifelong inquiry of exploring these questions and how the answers manifest in my home and kitchen environment. The culture of our kitchen environment is the space we create to nurture and care for ourselves and our family.

The food culture that I grew up with held a vein of richness that is still with me. My dad's garden never failed to produce an overflow of fresh zucchini/ courgette and squash. We lived in a town that was known for its rich history of fruit production. There were always trees to pick from, and the farm stands were brimming with each seasonal bounty. We purchased fruit by the box and made pies, cobbler, ice cream, and jam. My grandfather was a fisherman, and my father was an ocean diver. We always had a freezer full of fish and abalone, and many times throughout the year we had fresh seafood feasts, feeding loads of people the most delicious fruits of the sea.

My grandparents kept an annual tradition of harvesting wild mushrooms after the first spring and fall rains. I can still smell the mounds of garlic, onions, and mushrooms cooking in the enormous cast-iron frying pan on their stove. I remember them talking in amazement about how many helpings I could eat. I loved our family mushroom feasts. This celebration was a high point in our culinary culture, and everything about it is vivid in my mind as if it were yesterday. I can hear the sound of the knives on the wooden chopping board. I see the smiles on my grandparents' faces and hear the conversation and laughter of family and friends that came out of the woodwork for our holy day of mushroom gluttony. I was so awake and present for this vivacious celebration that centered on the pleasure and excitement of a single wild food.

When I was about fifteen years old, this tradition stopped. Development and overgrazing laid waste to the mushroom patches, and there just weren't as many mushrooms anymore. Even during the final years of my grandfather's life, he was still searching for mushroom patches to reappear. In the months before he died, we found a small patch of mushrooms together. We brought them home, and I watched him carefully, almost ceremoniously clean them so as not to waste a single piece. I remember sitting at his table, just he and I, humbly savoring our mushroom side dish. They were as delectable as ever, but what an impoverished relic of the fungal feasts of days gone by.

My mother went to work when I was in grade school. Prepackaged meals and processed snacks shared equal space at the table with food from the garden and the wild. Chocolate Pop-Tarts and Cap'n Crunch for breakfast, bologna on Wonder bread for lunch, and hot dog TV dinners for which my brother and I would beg. I can still picture the snack cupboard that we raided after school; it was full of Space Food Sticks, Cheez-Its, Fruit Loops, Ho Hos, and Ding Dongs.

Even though the junk food was plentiful, I was lucky to have had so much local fruit and wild foods to supplement the packaged meals. I grew up surrounded by seasonal food harvest traditions, which at specific times of the year shaped some of the culture of our household. My grandfather was a master ice cream maker and would concoct a batch to honor the onset of each seasonal fruit. It was most definitely the best ice cream on the planet. In the summer, there was always a cobbler or special jam from the peaches and apricots. Something had to be done with all the summer squash, and late summer meant filling the freezer with zucchini/courgette bread. Fall brought walnuts, which we gathered by the bucketful and candied for Christmas presents. Each food had a spice that went with it: nutmeg with peaches, orange zest with the zucchini/courgette breads, allspice with apricots, and cinnamon with apples. The turning of the seasons was clearly marked with flavors and aromas specific to each time of year.

What we create from the earth's harvest helps shape who we are and what we love. It sets the scope of our taste buds, priming our palate for which foods we crave and find comfort in. It provides our basic nourishment for a strong body and vibrant mind. For me, it also provided something that I can't really name. What was I fed as I sat in front of giant bags of walnuts, cracking and eating them with my grandparents? More than food was given to me at the table where we dined on fish that my dad taught me how to clean and cook. The need to harvest, create, and give away was embedded in my being. The ritual of picking blackberries in August is etched in my cells. I get a little cranky if the summer is coming to an end and I haven't made my annual pilgrimage to gorge at the blackberry patch and make blackberry pies. Each season holds a craving to honor what has ripened. Harvesting the abundance and sharing it brings me such joy.

When we don't grow up with seasonal food rituals, then it can be a challenge to know what to eat when. It is easy to fall into the trap of eating all foods all year around just because they are available in the grocery store. The strawberry festival is in April; what are the health and environmental implications of having access to a plateful of strawberries in December? Tomato tasting day is in August; do I really need fresh tomatoes on my sandwich in February? The perpetual deluge of advertisements tranquilizes any concern we may have about the chemicals and pollution involved in providing all fruits and vegetables during all seasons. We slip into eating what the media tells us to, not knowing what healthful, seasonal food really feels like in our body.

My grandparents still hunted and fished for wild foods. I got a taste of what it meant to harvest and eat wild, seasonal foods; but these were marginal events, and most of our food came from the store. How do those of us who grew up in households with a microwave and canned food make the change?

Wherever you live, there is or was a river of wild or cultivated local food and herb harvest for you to dive into. Get into the kitchen with your family and reclaim your food culture. When the apples are ripe, make apple cinnamon pie. When it is almond season, make herb-salted almonds. If you live in the heart of a city, befriend someone with a fruit tree or a planter box full of so much sage that one family can't possibly use it all, frequent local farmers' markets, or grow your own herbs in a window box or community garden. You will be inspired by the wonder of nature and how its gifts manifest in your kitchen as a way of life. It won't be long before the recipes on these pages evolve into the expression of your personal spice preferences and neighborhood gardens.

To this day, I love to find the trees that no one has harvested, glean the fruit that litters the ground, and transform this abundance of free food into jams and dried fruit for the lunch box. Summer's magnificence fills my shelf with a dozen herbal vinegars, and wild bay leaves gathered in autumn unfold their flavor into soups all year long. These small rituals guide our lives. I keep a watchful eye for what the earth has to offer, paying my respects by nourishing my body and soul with the harvest.

The knowledge of how to enjoy the earth's generosity to fortify ourselves and our loved ones is the inheritance of being human. If this tradition was lost in your family, you are in luck, because the harvest is still on. The earth hasn't stopped giving; we have just forgotten how to receive. Start by finding one local food or growing one herb in your backyard or window, see what you can make with it, and go from there. Interview some of the old-timers where you live. What local foods and herbs do they have stories about?

I try to grow as many of my own herbs and spices as the weather will permit. Herbal gardening has sculpted my life in so many ways. From the garden, I learn how to work in harmony with the seasons and seasonal transitions, the moon, and daily weather. It teaches me about life, death, decay, and regeneration, and it is the master teacher of change, the one thing that is certain in life. Working with the abundance of herbs and spices that come from the garden has deepened my ability to really feel gratitude. I am always so thankful and happy when the fertility of the garden allows me to give away a portion of the fortune to everyone who walks through my door.

Learning to garden, cook, and craft with herbs has been a very empowering process. The garden makes me work to find nonchemical solutions for weeds and pests. It is deeply fulfilling to use herbs and foods that help reduce reliance on chemicals, pesticides, and prescription and over-the-counter medications. Growing my own herbs and spices is my day-to-day way of increasing my health and well-being and living more harmoniously with and in right relationship to what is around me. As I write this book, I am forty-seven years old. I am just now beginning to feel that I have some assemblage of what it means to live in awareness of the natural systems that nurture and support my life. Each season, each year, nature's manifestation in my kitchen teaches me more.

The joyful journey of cooking with herbs is more than creating delicious and nutritious food; it is my pathway toward awareness of how to live in integrity on this earth. What does it mean to use whole foods and whole herbs as a lifestyle practice dedicated to healing? From the garden to the kitchen, we nurture life. We amass the health and wealth that benefits us for now and what is to come. The level of health we cultivate before we have babies is passed on to our children. What we eat and how well we digest contribute to the wellness and vitality of future generations. When you don't pollute your food and soil, then the actual place where the food is grown and used is in a more whole state. When you eat whole foods and herbs, you are accumulating health within your own body that is pledged to the unborn.

During the past century, our love affair with chemicals has shaped much of our lives. The food we eat, the medicine we take and the beverages we drink are processed and made with thousands of man-made chemicals. Our use of chemicals has come with many advantages and advancements, but our extended exposure to them has affected us in ways that we can't even begin to comprehend. The use of chemicals in our food production is not going to disappear, but let's just slow down a little. Let's use less, ban the chemicals that we already know are carcinogenic, look for nonchemical solutions, and err on the side of caution instead of limitless experimentation. Stop adding them to new products as if they have a right to be in every corner of our existence. We introduce new chemicals at the drop of a hat with very little understanding of their long-term effects on human and environmental health.

By indulging in chemicals this way, we have disrespected ourselves and the plants. The damage done by chemical fertilizers, pesticides, herbicides, and genetically engineered seeds is reflective of the loss of integrity in our relationship with the plants. We poison the plants and denature them to the point where we have not only shattered our covenant with the plant world but also our promise of the right to health for our children. We have polluted the air, soil, and water and all life that is sustained by these elements. The chemical methods of food production are degenerative in nature, wreaking havoc on our health and vitality. The rampant chemical waste poisons our body, our children's bodies, and the environment of those not yet conceived. I could get depressed if I dwell on the problem for too long, so I have learned to remain steadfast and focused on solutions: simple solutions that are attainable within our home and daily lives. The commitment to a lifestyle of using sustainable foods, healing herbs, and seasonal harvests is a choice that has broad-reaching implications in every aspect of our lives.

In recent years, there has been an explosion of awareness about the importance of local, organic, and sustainable food. Buying food from people we know and reducing our carbon footprint by shipping food a minimal distance to arrive at our dinner tables have become central issues. Sustainable care of home ailments is the next step in this groundswell of demand for organic food and a healthful lifestyle. Once the vegetable garden is established, it is just as easy to grow medicine as it is to grow food. Food and medicine cultivation are intricately related and grow side by side. There are a variety of medicinal herbs that attract beneficial insects to the garden. Many herbs pair well with vegetables and are cultivated as companion plants for successful organic vegetable gardening. Learning to use the herbs for health and wellness is an elemental component in the movement toward sustainability and reducing our dependence on chemicals and processed substances.

The current explosion of interest in sustainability practices is inspiring. There are vegetable gardens popping up in front yards everywhere. The surge of demand for local food and the profusion of organic vegetables that people are growing are nothing short of thrilling. We can feed ourselves good food and have a great time doing it. The cornucopia of herbs and vegetables are so prolific that we can't possibly use everything that the garden gives, so we share them with those around us. In the process, we talk to our neighbors more often, share recipes, celebrate the abundance with harvest festivals, and voila! Our culture begins to change shape. The conversations center on food, health, and the pleasure of our palate. Our bodies are stronger and our communities are more connected.

The garden and kitchen hold a central place of importance in the economy of your home and your family's health. How much does it cost when we get sick? How do you quantify the loss of basic herbal home care and cooking skills? How is the lack of home nourishment and wellness care reflected in wages, the gross national product, and the general well-being that is expressed as joy and passion for life? I have not been able to come up with a formula that can measure the personal, family, and community savings of a society that experiences increased vitality and greater health, but I know that it is significant. Just watch the financial and emotional ruin that happens when illness plagues a family member.

As the seasons go around and we notice which herbs grow well and promote health, we are assembling a base of body/earth knowledge that is empirical in nature. What is the best way to grow an herb? What are the most efficient harvesting methods, and what is the most effective way to preserve and dispense the spice cabinet? Direct perception guides us; we know what works through observation and experience. This is the knowledge that is accumulated over time and is passed on from generation to generation.

Many family home medicine lineages in the Western world were lost in the last several generations. We were mesmerized by the novelty and scientifically proven "superiority" of synthetic food and modern medicine. We cast our grandmothers' teas and herbal powders to the wind. I have often wondered how it must feel to a grandmother when her clan dismisses her ancient wisdom as an old wives' tale. This loss of ancestral food and medicine literacy is nothing short of tragic. I can't count the number of students that have come to class talking about their grandmothers' soups and herbal recipes that no one paid attention to and are now lost. Generations of observation of what herbs to use when and how to best prepare foods for optimal health traded for television advertisement medicine.

The current spice rack is a remnant of the wisdom of how to bring the earth's harvest into our homes to feed and keep our families well. It is the accumulation of thousands of years of experience all powdered and packaged into convenient little jars. Take a closer look at your spice rack. The herbs come from all over the world, having touched many hands; they carry the lineage of our ancestors' wisdom that using plants in our food helps keep us well.

What is the value of garnishing your meals with herbs that rid foods of pathogens and aid everyone at the table in digesting their food with ease? Who knows how many bellyaches, headaches, and colds are averted with the skill of the spice-wielding cook? "Eat, drink, and be merry" is a well-known saying, but it's hard to be merry unless what you eat is well spiced so you can digest it efficiently.

Our digestive process utilizes a significant amount of physical energy. When we eat packaged, chemical-laden foods, grouchiness sets in because our energy is siphoned into a discontented digestive system. When you are bogged down by foods that are difficult to assimilate, you don't participate as much in the pleasures that life has to offer. If you are going to devour a heavy meal, by all means look at the cornucopia of carminative digestive aids listed in this book. Don't go it alone; use herbs to help you digest your food! The spice cabinet is bursting with carminatives. It really is that simple. When you are supported in digesting your foods, you feel better, have more energy, and may even experience moments of exuberance and merriment after dinner.

*The Herbal Kitchen* is about the personal and communal joy of putting nature in your cupboard. It is about reclaiming the indispensable skill of using herbs to prevent sickness and take care of home ailments. Nurturing the life around us with the medicine from the kitchen revives our relationship with the plants and empowers our ability to understand our food, our body, and our relationship to sustaining healthy life.

For me, this information is much easier to embody when I share it with another person. Many of my students get together once a season and mix their oils, set up tinctures, and make seasonal foods and herbal remedies. Please don't put the recipes in this book on your to-do list as one more thing adding to the compression of overstimulation and activity. They should be a fun and relaxing opportunity to connect with those around you. What about a monthly herbal crafting get-together with even one other person who is interested in health?

Not everyone needs to be the cook, but all of us need someone in our life who is focused on what happens in the kitchen. I envision a culture where there is more meal sharing between families so that our food preparation can become more sustainable. Three families on one block can do meal trades, or group cooking days can produce meals for the week.

If you are overwhelmed with all of life's tasks, just begin by setting aside one afternoon a week for embracing food culture with your family. Like everyone else, our days are busy, but Wednesday afternoons from about three to five thirty, we play in the kitchen. We make pesto from explosions of basil, pies from summer apricots, juice from fall apples, and nut butter from the almond harvest, and pomegranate juice flows all winter long.

Once you establish a weekly food preparation ritual, it becomes habitual, and you miss it when it doesn't happen. It becomes the time to strain out the herbal oils, stock your pantry with herbal vinegars, whip up a new batch of herbed ghee, or make a special marinade for the evening meal. When there is a profusion of lavender in the garden, we store the seasonal harvest by making vinegars, oils, cordial, and many other condiments that enrich our meals. Ripe elderberries means black fingertips and a case of cordial. It is amazing what you can do in even a few hours a week. Set a time and create a rhythm, a food culture rhythm that will feed you and your household in more ways than you can name.

Stop and think right now about a structure that can help support you into really being able to incorporate more food preparation time into your life. It doesn't have to be a lot of time; look for a rhythm and find a way to be supported in that rhythm. It is a little bit like exercising: if you have a buddy, you are more likely to stick with it. This makes sense, because it is only a recent phenomenon that solitary people cook for just themselves or others. It is really not in our cellular memory to be alone in the kitchen. We always cooked in groups. Our current template of having one person as the main nurturer in a single-family household is really a new experiment. I don't know about you, but for me, cooking alone is a task. As soon as there is another person in the kitchen, it is fun!

Involve your children in using herbs. Provide them with simple ways to incorporate herbs into their food and cooking projects. Let them be in charge of garnishing their foods with herbs. We always have several herb sprinkles on the table that my son can use at any time. In classes I pass around a platter of little herb-filled bowls. People are usually inspired by the idea and, without much effort, put herbal condiments on their kitchen table for everyone to use. The feedback from introducing just this one little trick is amazing. People tell me how their kids are now using all kinds of herbal condiments and love sprinkling cinnamon on their oatmeal and rose hips on their rice. Children develop their taste preferences when they are young. Make it convenient for them to have opportunities to use herbs. Feed them now what you want them to eat throughout their lives. My son did not have one speck of processed sugar in his first year. At five years old, he has still never eaten boxed macaroni and cheese. He sprinkles herbs on almost all of his meals and picks his own peppermint tea when he has a bellyache.

Hopefully you will be inspired to fill your pantry to its holding capacity. Get ready to add more shelves to your kitchen storage area. Sacrifice a cabinet of dishes for more condiment space or remodel your kitchen just a little so it can house your herbal alchemy projects. What about all the bottles, jars, lids, strainers, teapots, and other paraphernalia? Build shelves above your cupboards; put standing cabinets in the garage, the spare bedroom, or a closet. Add a spice rack to the back of the kitchen door. When my husband and I went to look at the house we would live in for ten years, I said, "Oh yes, very nice, three bedrooms, two bathrooms, uh huh . . . but look at the granny flat, just behind the house! It is the perfect place for all my jars, bottles, and herbal infusions." It was heaven, an entire building for all of the infusing, fermenting, aging, soaking, macerating, percolating, mixing, marinating, and drying that takes place with my food and herbs. We have since moved to a place that doesn't have a second building, but the herbs now have their own bedroom, and they also dominate the garage.

Creating in your herbal kitchen is easy once you have your herbs and herbal blends organized and readily accessible to add to foods and beverages as often as possible. Keep a variety of herbal condiments next to your food preparation area as well as on your table. You can put powdered herbs in salt and pepper shakers or in tiny bowls with miniature spoons for sprinkling on your food. I am always looking to support our meals with herbs in as many ways as possible. Make up a half dozen oils and vinegars and have them on hand to support you in the kitchen. Some days you may not have a creative flow going, or your garden isn't producing yet, or you didn't get to the market for fresh ingredients. Let the herbal oils, vinegar, ghee, and sprinkles give you a hand. Incorporate herbs into your oils, vinegars, honey, and butter, and soon your food will encompass gourmet seasonings that taste delicious and keep your family healthy.

# PART TWO

# Fifty Healing Herbs and Spices

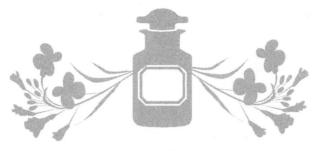

CHAPTER 2

# Herbal Kitchen Materia Medica

"Materia medica" simply means the materials of medicine that you use in your household. The plants we settle with depend on from whom we've learned, where we live, and what is accessible. It is very important to have proper identification of any plant that you use. If you are not 100 percent sure about a plant, don't pick it. Many plants are poisonous, and working with fresh herbs requires that you have complete accuracy. Many of the herbs discussed have stronger actions when used therapeutically in larger doses than suggested in this book. The recipes and suggestions in *The Herbal Kitchen* are primarily for culinary use. Sprinkle and dollop your way to good health!

Normally the word "herb" refers to the green leafy part of a plant that is often used fresh. Spices are normally categorized as the roots, seeds, bark, and berries that are dried and found in your spice cabinet. In the study of botanical medicine, all parts of a plant that are medicinal are lumped into a single category under the word "herbs." So, if they have medicinal qualities, spices are also called herbs. "Herb" is a general term for all parts of plants that are used to heal. Throughout the book, the words "herb" and "spice" are used interchangeably.

In the following materia medica, many of the "projects" listed are discussed in later chapters. There aren't recipes for all the projects, though. The projects listed are simply suggestions for how you might want to use each herb. Any oil uses in this book are for infused herbal oils as described in chapter 9. This book does not cover the uses of essential oils.

**COMMON NAME:** **allspice**

**BOTANICAL NAME:** *Pimenta dioica*

**PART USED:** **berry**

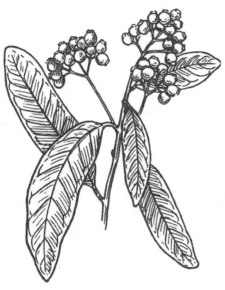

**GARDENING TIPS:** Allspice grows in tropical climates and is widely cultivated in Jamaica.

**PROPERTIES:** anesthetic, antibacterial, antioxidant, antispasmodic, antiviral, carminative, circulatory stimulant, rubefacient

**USES:** It is time to expand the horizons of allspice use beyond the ingredient lists for pumpkin pie and mulled cider. Found in almost every cupboard, this warming and pungent spice is a vitamin supplement and medicine chest packed into a small berry. Allspice is high in vitamins and minerals including calcium, iron, and manganese. Allspice fights off colds and flu, calms menstrual cramps, settles upset stomachs, and enhances the delivery of nutrients in the body.

Sprinkle a mixture of cinnamon and allspice on your toast or make allspice juniper berry oil and drizzle it on potatoes and baked root vegetables. Add a little powdered allspice to any flour mix for pancakes, muffins, cookies/biscuits, and bread or put a dash in your hot chocolate. I make a scrumptious wheat-free almond cake that has allspice and nutmeg in the almond flour. Allspice is also a staple spice in sauerkraut and pickled vegetables.

Allspice is a great digestive aid, helping to lighten the load and assisting in the breakdown of heavy foods. Just because you consume something doesn't mean it can be processed into healthy cells. Large food molecules have to be split into smaller, more soluble molecules in order to pass through the cell membrane. This is no easy task. Herbs and spices are in your cupboard to assist your body in the daily digestion of other life-forms into your cells.

When you are satisfied with your allspice endeavors in the kitchen, wander into the bathroom and make an allspice foot bath for cold and achy feet. You'll soon give it the name all-purpose allspice when you experience the luxury of an allspice body scrub. Mix 2 tablespoons (5 g) powdered allspice with ½ cup (120 ml) olive oil and use it as a body scrub for sore joints and cold extremities. If you want to get even more creative with this little black berry, soak it in some witch hazel for a month, strain it out of the witch hazel, and then use the witch hazel as an aftershave. It has the perfect smell for a manly aftershave, and it tightens and tones the skin after shaving. A little bit of allspice goes a long way in spicing up your life.

**PROJECTS:** herbal waters, herbal drinks, herbal smoothies, herbal honey, herbal vinegar, herbal cordial, herbal oil, herbal ghee, herbal sprinkle, herbal bath and foot soak

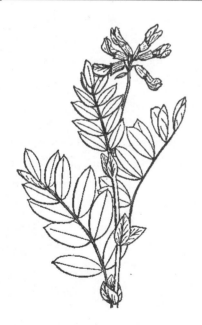

**COMMON NAME: astragalus**

**BOTANICAL NAME:** *Astragalus membranaceus*

**PART USED: root**

**GARDENING TIPS:** Astragalus requires well-drained, sandy soil and lots of sun. It is a hardy plant that withstands frost and can survive with little water.

**PROPERTIES:** adaptogen, antibacterial, anti-inflammatory, antioxidant, antiviral, demulcent, tonic

**USES:** Astragalus has a very pleasant taste that blends well into soups and grain dishes. We add astragalus to just about any grain, bean, or soup that is prepared during the fall and winter. Astragalus root that can be purchased in the store is precut into long, thin wedges that look like tongue depressors. Just throw two or three of these flattened sticks into any soup that you make. Add them at the beginning of the soup preparation and leave the sticks in the pot until the soup is finished. Don't serve them; let them continue to steep in the broth until the soup or stew is gone. When you cook grains such as rice, barley, or quinoa, throw a couple of astragalus sticks in with the grain and water and let the root steep during the cooking process. Remove the astragalus before serving the grains.

Autumn is a good time of year to eat and drink astragalus, as it builds the immune system in preparation for cold and flu season. Enjoy the mild taste of the tea or put it in soups and grains. Astragalus is antiviral and strengthens the body's resistance to sickness. Not only does astragalus inhibit viral growth, it also enhances the immune system on many different levels. It increases the activity of natural killer cells and the overall ability of the body to scavenge pathogenic bacteria. It can increase vitality during the recuperative phase after an illness. When your local school shuts its doors for the week due to a flu scare, herbs that provide extra support for the immune system become even more important. This amazing root also helps to strengthen the lungs and is a great tonic for people with a propensity for respiratory problems during the winter.

This valuable medicine increases resilience and stamina and invigorates the vital force. Astragalus is known to restore energy levels in healthy people. It has an enlivening and rejuvenating effect, counteracting the ravages of stress. This woody, sweet-tasting root is often used to revive immune function after chemotherapy. I love the gentle yet powerful nature of astragalus. It does so many things for us and is so easy to cook with. I hope you are inspired to try it!

**PROJECTS:** herbal drinks, herbal honey, herbal ghee, herbal sprinkle, herbal bath and foot soak

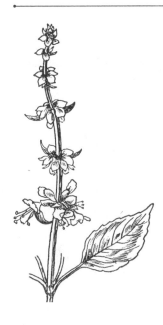

**COMMON NAME: basil**

**BOTANICAL NAME: *Ocimum basilicum***

**PART USED: leaf and flower**

**GARDENING TIPS:** Basil likes full summer sun and average water. Pinching off the flower heads encourages larger leaf growth. Basil dies after the first frost but loves the full glory of summer. When the heat of summer peaks, you know it is time to fill the freezer with pesto.

**PROPERTIES:** antibacterial, antispasmodic, antiviral, carminative, nervine

**USES:** The warming, aromatic constituents of basil help to calm the nervous system; settle the stomach; clear the mind; and fight off coughs, colds, flu, and allergies. The magnitude of basil's healing endeavors are reflected in the hundreds of therapeutic applications of this leafy green companion. Basil is known as the destroyer of phlegm. When you consider the number of ailments that are provoked by excess phlegm—from allergies to asthma to colds—you begin to understand the breadth of basil's virtue.

Basil is most commonly thought of as part of the tomato sauce or pasta dish, but a cup of basil tea works wonders for almost any digestive complaint. Basil tea relieves stomach cramps and spasms, nausea, gas, and constipation. That must be why it is a primary ingredient in pasta dishes: so you can eat more pasta! Basil doesn't qualify for the world's best-tasting tea, but it is not so bad, especially when you find out what it can do for your stomach. Add a little honey to your basil tea and the next time you eat a heavy pasta meal, drink a cup. You won't feel like just passing out after dinner, and instead you'll still be able to think straight and actually feel like socializing with the people you dined with.

Dry some of basil's bountiful summer harvest to use in winter sauces and dressings. I dry a lot of basil every year and add it to whatever gets cooked up in the slow cooker during the cold months. Another simple way to store your fresh basil is to put 1 cup (30 g) basil leaves and 1½ cups (360 ml) olive oil in the blender and blend it until you have a nice paste. Freeze this paste in containers and cook with it throughout the rest of the year.

Eating more basil in the late summer and early fall helps fend off sinus and bronchial congestion during the winter. If you suffer from any sickness that is exasperated by phlegm, eat more basil! For many people, certain foods such as dairy or wheat can cause more mucus. It is usually a good idea to eliminate foods from the diet that cause overt mucus production, but eating basil may help you reduce your reaction to them.

Basil is antibacterial and antiviral, making it a helpful remedy for the common cold and flu. If you are prone to bronchitis or chest colds, dry some of your basil, store it in a jar, and drink the tea several times a week as a preventive remedy. It warms the body, clears out the bugs, and sharpens the mind. In the middle of winter when you are feeling cold, dark, damp, and depressed, break out your stash of dried basil or frozen pesto and let it infuse your day with a little warmth and summer sunshine.

**PROJECTS:** herbal waters, herbal drinks, herbal smoothies, herbal honey, herbal vinegar, herbal cordial, herbal oil, herbal ghee, herbal pesto, herbal sprinkle, herbal bath and foot soak

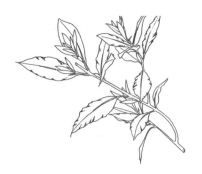

**COMMON NAME: bay leaf**

**BOTANICAL NAME:** *Laurus nobilis*

**PART USED: leaf**

**GARDENING TIPS:** Bay laurel is a slow-growing tree that needs to be pruned into a shrub or it will grow into a very, very large tree. They can grow to be 50 feet (15 meters)

tall, so if you don't have enough space, keep them cut back. Even a small bay tree is a pleasure to have around. I love being able to pick fresh leaves throughout the year for my beans and sauces. Bay likes full sun and moderate winters. It can withstand some frost and likes occasional watering. If you live in a climate with more severe winters, grow the bay in a pot and bring it inside for the winter.

**PROPERTIES:** anthelmintic, antibacterial, antifungal, astringent, carminative, emmenagogue, expectorant, rubefacient

**USES:** Have you ever been at a potluck dinner and gone from wondering what was the secret ingredient in the soup to wondering what is making you feel so ill? Many years ago, I learned from my teacher, Vasant Lad, that it is exactly situations like these that you don't sit around and wait for the body to resolve. It takes too much energy to fight off food pathogens and digest poorly cooked foods. Get some help, and the sooner the better. When you first realize you have been gastronomically assaulted, break out the bay leaves. Drink a cup of bay leaf tea, take a short walk, then take a little rest so your body can focus on the task at hand. The pungent and warming bay leaf will activate your digestive capacity, relieve your gut distress, and help you actually absorb some nutrients from the meal.

Bay leaves are a great additive to beans, grains, soups, and sauces for invigorating digestion and supporting healthy elimination. Enhanced absorption improves your overall health. How well you absorb your nutrients dictates the quality of what you use to build your cells. You are only as healthy as what you digest. Even the healthiest of foods becomes toxic if you don't assimilate and eliminate properly. When we don't assimilate nutrients well, our vitality and passion for life begins to wane. Adding digestive herbs to food can literally make people feel happier and more enthusiastic about life.

Bay leaves have a long history of being used in European games and festivals. When I got married, bay leaves were the most prolific treasure in our garden, so we dried it, packaged them in bottles with an attractive label, and gave them away as wedding favors. I loved the idea of people being reminded of the beauty and joy of our ceremony as they opened the jar of bay leaves.

Before I even knew that herbal medicine existed, I had heard of the winners of ancient Greek games being crowned with a wreath of bay laurel leaves. Beaming with a lineage steeped in fame and glory, bay must be doing something victorious in my stew. No spaghetti sauce would be complete without bay leaf, and there are always a few floating around in my slow cooker stews. Put dried bay leaf into storage containers of flour and grains to repel insects. Make sure you add a bay leaf or two to the water when cooking grains and beans. They work wonders on the digestibility of beans. Be sure to remove the leaf before serving, as it is a possible choking hazard.

**PROJECTS:** herbal vinegar, herbal cordial, herbal oil, herbal ghee, herbal sprinkle, herbal bath and foot soak

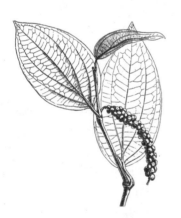

**COMMON NAME:** **black pepper**

**BOTANICAL NAME:** *Piper nigrum*

**PART USED:** **seed**

**GARDENING TIPS:** Black pepper is the seed of a vine that is cultivated in tropical locations around the world.

**PROPERTIES:** anthelmintic, antibacterial, anti-inflammatory, antioxidant, aperient, carminative, circulatory stimulant, expectorant, rubefacient

**USES:** Of all the herbs that have traveled the globe to enliven our palate and improve our health, pepper is the herb that has been elevated to "every table in America" status. The omnipresence of this spice is astonishing; you find it conveniently packed and ready to use everywhere you turn: in airline meals, the fast-food drive-through, packaged lunches, fine dining establishments, outdoor concerts, hotel meeting rooms, cafeterias, gas stations, and truck stop diners. We have come to expect our provision of pepper to be replenished everywhere we go; it is one of our inherent rights. Watch the chaos develop if a restaurant runs out of pepper for its customers during lunch hour!

This isn't the first time in history that pepper has captivated the masses. This little black seed has been used to pay taxes, wages, rent, bribes, dowries, and ransoms, and its value as a commodity has been the impetus for ocean voyages and wars. Why? Because pepper truly is an extraordinary spice. Pepper keeps people happy. It is the emperor of digestive aids. As one of nature's strongest digestive stimulants, pepper bolsters the healing process in a number of belly complaints: bloating, belching, burping, farting, constipation, distension, indigestion, nausea, stomachache, and stomach cramps. What does pepper do for you?

Pepper stimulates gastric juices that help with the digestion of rich foods. Blue cheese dressing? Add pepper. Cream-filled clam chowder? Add pepper. Rich hollandaise sauce or fish and chips with tartar sauce? Definitely add pepper. The standard American diet tends to be overloaded with an excess of poor-quality meat, denatured oil, sugar, unhealthful table salt, not to mention all the pesticides, chemicals, food preservatives, and dyes. Think of pepper as a first aid remedy for the average American diet.

Pepper's pungent and heating nature facilitates dispersal of nutrients throughout the body. It also dissolves mucus, drains chronic sinus congestion, and helps you to digest and absorb what you consume. There are lots of recipes throughout this book that include pepper, so it can infiltrate your food in a myriad of creative ways. Drink a mixture of ¼ teaspoon (½ g) powdered black pepper, 1 teaspoon (8 ml) of honey, and 1 cup (250 ml) hot water to get rid of a wet cough. Make a pepper-thyme honey to disperse lung mucus and assist poor circulation. Use pepper ghee to improve weak digestion, and put pepper in your culinary oils to enhance the assimilation of nutrients in meat dishes. You probably already use pepper; now you know more about why you do.

**PROJECTS:** herbal honey, herbal vinegar, herbal cordial, herbal oil, herbal ghee, herbal pesto, herbal sprinkle, herbal bath and foot soak

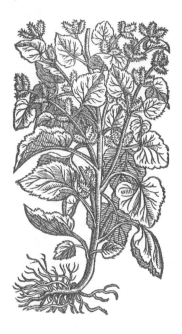

**COMMON NAME: burdock**

**BOTANICAL NAME:** *Arctium lappa*

**PART USED: root**

**GARDENING TIPS:** This herb grows wild in many places in the United States. It is invasive and easy to grow. It doesn't mind poor, compacted soil or frosty winters. Burdock throws off millions of seeds and easily reseeds itself. It is somewhat drought tolerant but needs occasional watering during hot months. Burdock has honorably claimed weed status where we live.

**PROPERTIES:** alterative, antibacterial, antifungal, anti-inflammatory, aperient, carminative, cholagogue, demulcent, emollient, nutritive, vulnerary

**USES:** Burdock root is a cooling, nutrient-dense herbal food. It is an edible vegetable that is very popular in Japanese cuisine, in which it is known as gobo. This mineral-rich root goes into most of my soup stocks. I also add it to rice and other grains as they are cooking. Drink burdock tea or sauté it with other root vegetables. Put a stick of burdock in a pot of beans as you simmer them and take it out just before serving the beans.

This revitalizing root is teeming with healing properties. Scientists continue to examine its anticancer and antitumor effects. Saturated with minerals, it is high in calcium, phosphorus, iron, chromium, and magnesium. Its nutritive and demulcent properties give burdock a restorative quality that nourishes the body and soothes the skin. Burdock root helps to resolve acne, eczema, psoriasis, boils, and most inflammatory skin conditions.

We have external skin that protects the outside of the body, and we have an internal mucous membrane skin that lines the inside of the body from the mouth to the anus. The internal mucous membrane can become weak and inflamed, allowing for undesirable bacteria and undigested foods to enter the blood. Demulcent herbs protect the internal mucous membranes of the digestive tract and help prevent the inflammatory conditions that plague that part of the body. Burdock's demulcent capability provides a protective shield for the mucous membrane, soothing, coating, and lubricating to bolster your health.

Burdock root is also known for its aptitude in supporting sluggish digestion and relieving lymph stagnation. Burdock helps alleviate lymph congestion, including swollen glands and benign lumps. Put burdock into your bath to soothe dry, irritated skin or put it in your soup to lubricate and protect your intestines. Burdock tea has a somewhat mild and sweet flavor, so you can add the tea to smoothies and fruit drinks. Burdock and dandelion vinegar makes a tasty and nutritious addition to vinaigrette dressings and soup stocks.

**PROJECTS:** herbal drinks, herbal honey, herbal vinegar, herbal cordial, herbal ghee, herbal sprinkle, herbal bath and foot soak

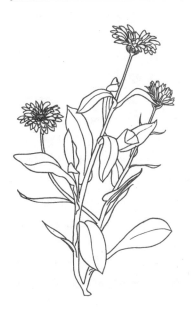

**COMMON NAME: calendula**

**BOTANICAL NAME:** *Calendula officinalis*

**PART USED: flower**

**GARDENING TIPS:** The more you pick calendula flowers, the more they grow. I like this kind of plant! Calendula will grow in full sun but also does well with some shade. It survives with little watering, and I have even seen it naturalize without any water except the rainfall. However, if you want luscious, large flowers to eat and drink, it needs moderate water or a regular influx of moist, coastal air.

**PROPERTIES:** anti-inflammatory, antispasmodic, antiviral, bitter tonic, demulcent, cholagogue, emollient, vulnerary

**USES:** Sprinkle the fresh flowers onto just about anything you eat, such as salads, sandwiches, and tacos. Add dried calendula flowers to soup and broths. Drink the golden petals in tea, include them in your cordials, and add them to smoothies.

The beautiful sunshine-colored petals of the calendula flower are a first-rate skin healer. Eat or drink them to heal inflammatory digestive conditions or infuse them into your bathwater for remedying skin irritations. The vulnerary effects of calendula soothe and repair acute and chronic skin problems, alleviating acne, swelling, cold sores, tissue trauma, slow-healing skin cuts, bruises, abrasions, sprains, psoriasis, eczema, hemorrhoids, and bug bites. For a reviving foot bath, mix calendula and lavender together, soak your feet, and release the strain and stress from your body.

When you think of calendula, besides being enamored with its vibrant color, think of wound healing and tissue regeneration throughout the entire body. It enhances the growth of damaged skin cells and reduces injury recovery time. Calendula also soothes the throat, making it a specifically useful ingredient in a gargle or mouthwash for sensitive gums.

Calendula encourages the healthy flow of lymph throughout the body. The lymph system supplies oxygen and nutrients to cells and tissue. It distributes immunity and forms a network throughout the body that removes waste and pathogens. Stagnant lymph sets the stage for a profusion of ailments. Motivate your lymph and pamper yourself with calendula body oil and calendula baths. Keep your lymph moving with exercise, stretching, and calendula flowers.

Calendula blooms in my garden all year long. It finds its way into my house just about every week of the year. I love what it does for my skin in the bathtub and I like to impress guests by garnishing any hors d'oeuvre, salad, or main dish with the fresh yellow petals.

**PROJECTS:** herbal waters, herbal drinks, herbal smoothies, herbal vinegar, herbal cordial, herbal oil, herbal ghee, herbal pesto, herbal sprinkle, herbal bath and foot soak

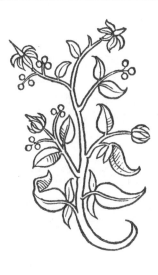

**COMMON NAME: cardamom**

**BOTANICAL NAME:** *Eletarria cardamomum*

**PART USED: fruit**

**GARDENING TIPS:** It helps to live in a sub-tropical forest to grow this spice.

**PROPERTIES:** antibacterial, anticatarrh, anti-inflammatory, antispasmodic, carminative, cholagogue, decongestant, expectorant, nervine, tonic

**USES:** Look at your tongue in the mirror. If you have a thick white coating, it usually means that there is stagnation in your digestive system, and cardamom may be a good herb for you to use more of in your cooking. Cardamom is the perfect herb for moving out congestion, dampness, and mucus. Cardamom has decongesting properties that help to clear mucus from the digestive tract and the lungs. If you have respiratory mucus that creates wet, phlegmy coughs, do I have some great recipes for you!

Purchase whole cardamom pods, which consist of little back seeds tucked into a green papery cover. When you are ready to use the seeds, discard the green pod. Mix powdered cardamom, cinnamon, and clove into honey. Make a tea by adding 1 tablespoon (23 ml) of this honey to 1 cup (250 ml) hot water. This is a delicious remedy that alleviates long-standing wet lung conditions and over time can help dissolve the thick white tongue coating. Like many culinary spices, cardamom is carminative, which means it increases the flow of oxygen and blood to the digestive tract, enhancing digestive function in one way or another. If you eat well but experience gas and bloating, you aren't digesting well. Cardamom helps relieve gas and indigestion and assists you in converting food into something your body can use. It helps with irritable bowel problems and is restorative to the digestive tract.

Digestive aids are one of the most valuable medicines from the plant world. Digesting what you eat uses up a lot of your daily vitality. When you take herbs to support digestion, they help save your energy so that you have a little more zip for other things in your life. Have you ever just felt like lying down after a big holiday meal? That is because the digestion process is draining all the energy you have. Adding cardamom and other carminative herbs to your holiday meal can help everyone stay awake after dinner! You may not always eat holiday feast proportions, but any heavy meal needs the helping hand of carminatives.

Sprinkle the warmth of cardamom into foods that can cause congestion like bananas, yogurt, ice cream, and frozen smoothies. Add a dash to all mixes for pancakes, waffles, scones, and muffins. I like to make herbal chai with extra cardamom and drink it in the afternoon as a pick-me-up instead of coffee. The cardamom in chai helps with headaches caused by indigestion, and its strong antibacterial properties ward off colds and flu. Cardamom-ginger oil makes the perfect massage oil for people who have heavier constitutions and need massage to help with circulation and energy flow.

**PROJECTS:** herbal waters, herbal drinks, herbal smoothies, herbal honey, herbal cordial, herbal oil, herbal ghee, herbal sprinkle, herbal bath and foot soak

---

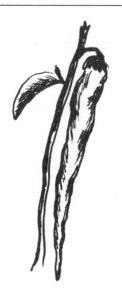

**COMMON NAME: cayenne**

**BOTANICAL NAME:** *Capsicum spp.*

**PART USED: fruit**

**GARDENING TIPS:** Cayenne is cultivated in a variety of different climates. It likes even moistness in the soil and a long, hot summer.

**PROPERTIES:** alterative, analgesic, anesthetic, anti-inflammatory, antioxidant, antispasmodic, circulatory stimulant, hemostat, nutritive, rubefacient, vulnerary

**USES:** Cayenne peppers vary considerably in heat, which is measured in heat units ranging from 0 at sweet and mild to a tongue-blistering 5,000. Capsicums originated in South America and spread across the globe, with each culture hybridizing the pepper, resulting in a broad range of flavors and heat quotients. There are lots and lots and lots of different kinds of capsicum. When you grow them yourself, you realize that even when you plant the same kind of pepper, its flavor varies from year to year. For the sake of our conversation, paprika is a mild and sweet pepper, cayenne is the hot and pungent pepper, and there are several varieties in between to explore.

Cayenne is antibacterial, gets rid of cold and flu, dissolves mucus and congestion, reduces nerve pain, and stops bleeding. It is a medicinal herb that not only intensifies the flavor of foods but also augments the delivery of the nutrients and medicinal qualities of other herbs. Cayenne dilates surface capillaries, stimulating blood circulation and the delivery of oxygen and nutrients throughout the body. It increases the blood supply to capillaries in the lining of the brain and helps with headaches and mental fog. Everyone has probably experienced the sinus-draining effect of cayenne. One bite, and suddenly tears come streaming down your cheeks and it seems that liquid is pouring out of every orifice. Cayenne can clear out congestion, colds, runny noses, and headaches. It is truly a head-clearing herb.

Cayenne is well known for its pain-relieving faculties. It contains capsaicin, which is found in several topical pain reliever creams. Capsaicin causes the body to release substance P, which is a pain messenger to the nervous system. Eventually substance P becomes temporarily depleted and the pain is diminished. Apply cayenne-infused oil to arthritic joints, sore muscles, and any nerve pain, including shingles.

Here is a cayenne remedy that you will remember. If you cut your finger in the kitchen, first rinse the cut with slightly warm water and let it bleed for a little bit under tepid running water. If you need to go to the hospital, by all means, do so, but if you have a superficial cut, rinse it and then cake it with cayenne. I know what your first thought is. We had many opportunities to try this remedy with minor knife cuts in herbal cooking classes, so I have watched a number of people go from an adamant "No way" to "Wow, this is miraculous." The cayenne stings for just a moment, and then it stops the bleeding, takes away the pain, and disinfects the wound. It is an herbal treatment that most professional cooks know about. You can wrap up the cut and keep on cooking if you have to.

If you ingest something that had way to much cayenne for your liking and your nose feels as if it is about ready to burn off the front of your face, the first thing people often do is reach for the ice water—don't do that unless you like pain. Water makes the heat worse. Eat some fat, like milk, yogurt, a piece of cheese, or some buttered bread; these foods will stop the flesh-piercing burn. Be careful not to touch your eyes after working with cayenne.

**PROJECTS:** herbal honey, herbal vinegar, herbal cordial, herbal oil, herbal ghee, herbal pesto, herbal sprinkle, herbal bath and foot soak

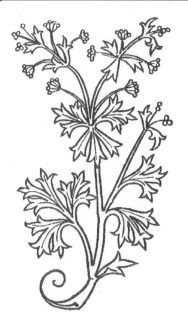

**COMMON NAME: celery seed**

**BOTANICAL NAME:** *Apium graveolens*

**PART USED: seed**

**GARDENING TIPS:** Celery seed is the seed of the celery vegetable that is chopped into soups and potato salad. It is a vegetable crop that likes plenty of water and rich soil.

**PROPERTIES:** antibacterial, antifungal, anti-inflammatory, antioxidant, bitter tonic, carminative, diuretic, emmenagogue, expectorant, nervine

**USES:** Celery seed has a reputation for easing a broad range of ailments including anxiety, arthritis, bronchitis, colds and flu, colic, cough, gas, gout, heartburn, indigestion, irritability, menstrual cramps, muscle spasms, nausea, restlessness, and skin problems. Are you inspired to pull the celery seed from the back of the cupboard? It is much more than a tomato juice seasoning for Sunday morning Bloody Marys!

Celery seed has a pungent, bitter flavor that goes well with creamy soups and dressings. Celery seed adds a salty tang to herbal salt substitutes. It lends an aromatic note to eggs, fish, stews, and potatoes. Celery seed and fennel seed sprinkle adds a nice finishing touch to potato salad and sauerkraut. I like to make a ghee with celery seed, fennel, ginger, and coriander for baked or sautéed vegetables.

The bitterness of celery seed makes it an effective herb for activating the digestive process. When you experience the bitter taste of any bitter herb or food, it stimulates the flow of gastric juices. Stress, hurried or emotional eating, eating when angry or upset, eating in the car or in front of the computer— all of these common habits inhibit the flow of gastric juices and curb digestive function. The bitter taste of herbs like celery seed or dandelion greens can help compensate for a compromised digestive system while we are getting around to creating a lifestyle of eating in a more calm and relaxed environment.

Celery seed improves circulation to the joints and muscles and clears stagnation that can exacerbate arthritic conditions. It has a stimulating and soothing affect on the stomach and alleviates muscle cramps and spasms. This itsy-bitsy, teeny-tiny seed is a decongestant for the respiratory system and dispels mucus from the lungs. Celery seed calms the nerves and makes a useful tea for bringing on a delayed menstruation. It also helps alleviate the fluid retention often associated with menstruation. Are you convinced yet to use more celery seed in your seasoning?

**PROJECTS:** herbal honey, herbal vinegar, herbal cordial, herbal ghee, herbal pesto, herbal sprinkle, herbal bath and foot soak

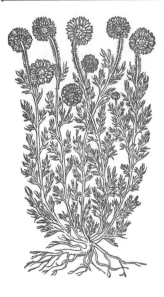

**COMMON NAME:** chamomile

**BOTANICAL NAME:** *Matricaria recutita* (German chamomile)

**PART USED:** flower

**GARDENING TIPS:** For the best results, plant chamomile in full sun. Keep it moderately watered in well-drained soil. This herb is easy to grow, and the quality of home grown-chamomile is far superior to anything you can purchase.

**PROPERTIES:** antibacterial, anticatarrh, anti-inflammatory, antispasmodic, carminative, cholagogue, nervine, vulnerary

**USES:** Chamomile is famous for its ability to relax and calm the nervous system even during the most stressful times. It helps with irritability, insomnia, and restlessness, and is the herb of choice for relaxing after a stressful day.

Chamomile is the universal home remedy for tension that manifests in a myriad of ways. Chamomile lavender massage oil relaxes rock-hard muscles, chamomile-fennel tea settles an upset stomach caused by anxiety and exasperated by stress. Chamomile-cinnamon tea will relax the uterus and alleviate painful menstrual cramps. Chamomile-ginger preparations reduce stress-induced inflammation that creates headaches, heartburn, gastritis, and stomach irritations. There is a saying: "If you don't know what to do, try chamomile."

Chamomile is a great herb for kids, but the tea is a little bitter, so make a chamomile honey to have on hand for an upset tummy. It relieves gas, soothes indigestion, and will take care of most stomachaches. Baths are the perfect way to dispense chamomile to children. Teach your children to bathe with herbs as early in their lives as possible. My son walks through the garden and fills his shirt full of herbs for his evening bath. Chamomile and rose petals are his favorite bathing herbs. He is a highly active boy, so chamomile has been a good choice for helping him to find balance. I think of chamomile as a quieting herb, having the same effect as a sweetly sung lullaby.

Vulnerary herbs heal the skin, and chamomile is a vigorous skin-repairing herb for both internal and external skin tissue. It quickens healing for scrapes, cuts, and abrasions. It soothes and softens red itchy skin, reduces healing time after burns, and promotes tissue repair in general.

Chamomile's bitter flavor has long been employed to facilitate digestion. There are numerous aperitifs formulated in Europe that tout chamomile's benevolence, including vermouth, the popular fortified wine. Drinking a small amount of bitter aperitif is a customary practice that stems from time-tested health wisdom that a little sip of bitter helps the dinner go down.

Chamomile is in the ragweed family. Use with caution if you have an allergic sensitivity to plants in the ragweed family.

**PROJECTS:** herbal water, herbal drinks, herbal smoothies, herbal honey, herbal vinegar, herbal cordial, herbal oil, herbal ghee, herbal bath and foot soak

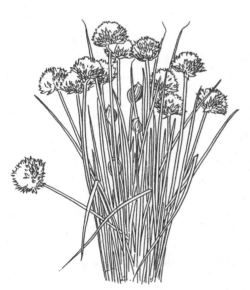

**COMMON NAME: chive**

**BOTANICAL NAME:** *Allium schoenoprasum*

**PART USED: leaf**

**GARDENING TIPS:** Chives like full sun or partial shade and well-drained soil with moderate watering. They tolerate frost, and once established they just grow and grow, and eventually you have to divide the clumps and plant them in other areas of the garden. This herb can sometimes take its time getting started, but it is worth the wait, because fresh chives are a cook's comrade.

**PROPERTIES:** anthelmintic, antibacterial, antioxidant, carminative, circulatory stimulant

**USES:** Old European lore talks about hanging bundles of chives in the home to ward off evil spirits. Well, chives do chase away colds that can feel pretty evil sometimes. Like garlic, chives contain the antiseptic properties of sulfur, which exterminate bugs that don't belong in your body. Chives are in the same family as onions and garlic, which are well known for their therapeutic actions. Chives boast many of the same healing benefits celebrated in garlic. Some of the most notable are stimulating circulation and lowering blood pressure.

Chives contain plenty of vitamins A and C and are a powerful antioxidant. Antioxidant herbs help protect your cells from damage caused by unstable molecules known as free radicals. Along with being a natural by-product of the body's metabolic process, free radical damage increases with exposure to stress, pesticides, and environmental toxins. Free radicals can increase the risk of heart disease, cancer, and premature aging. Eat more chives to help mop up the free radicals.

Chives are a cold and flu remedy that can easily be included in everyday meals. Take advantage of the abundance of antibacterial properties and use plenty of chives during cold and flu season. My husband reserves chives for that special place on top of the sour cream and butter in his baked potato, but they are one of the most prolific herbs in my garden, so I put them on everything. Their peppery onion flavor adds a zing to just about any savory dish. Often dried chives take the place of salt in our dinner. Their high vitamin C content is another reason to use them as a general condiment.

The secret to getting the highest nutritive value from your chives is to avoid cooking them. Add chives to vinegar, oil, ghee, pesto, and dried sprinkles or garnish your food with fresh or dried chives just before eating. We have a condiment shaker on the kitchen table that contains dried chives and sesame seeds; it is a delicious sprinkle for eggs and salads.

**PROJECTS:** herbal honey, herbal vinegar, herbal cordial, herbal oil, herbal ghee, herbal pesto, herbal sprinkle

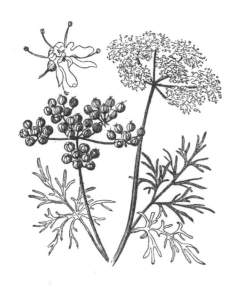

**COMMON NAME: cilantro (also known as Italian parsley or fresh coriander)**

**BOTANICAL NAME:** *Coriandrum sativum*

**PART USED: leaf**

**GARDENING TIPS:** Cilantro likes a moist place in the center of the garden with partial shade. It does not tolerate frost or high temperatures. It likes a little sun and a lot of moisture. If it gets too hot and the cilantro leaf fades away, it is okay, because the seed phase supplies you with coriander. This plant gives you two medicines for the price of one.

**PROPERTIES:** antibacterial, antifungal, anti-inflammatory, antispasmodic, carminative, nutritive

**USES:** Cilantro is also called Italian parsley or fresh coriander. When the plant goes to seed, the seeds are the spice known as coriander. Cilantro is the young leaves of the coriander plant. Chopped cilantro is easily added as a garnish to tacos, spring rolls, salads, soups, rice dishes, stir-fries, and fish. Whenever you go to a restaurant that has a salsa bar, heap on an extra helping of cilantro. This delicious green herb is nothing short of a healing ally.

The pleasant taste of cilantro fades quickly with heat. The frilly leaves wilt into nothing if you cook them. Cilantro really is best added raw as a garnish or put into sauces for foods that have already been cooked. I love minced cilantro in salads. We also use cilantro pesto instead of mayonnaise on our sandwiches. You really don't need basil for your pesto if you have cilantro.

Many spices are warming and heating to the body, whereas cilantro is cooling. People are often already overheated with stress and toxic foods, and the addition of lots of hot spices can be aggravating. Cilantro is a common ingredient in salsa, and it is made into condiment sauces in Indian cuisine because it helps to temper the harshness of spicy foods. What is nice about cilantro is that it is balancing to all body types, whether you are a hot or cold person, cilantro is good for you.

Cilantro aids digestion; it calms excess "heat" in the body and can relieve nausea. This tender leafy herb relieves headaches, gas, bloating, and upset stomachs. Cilantro is the perfect herb to eat throughout the summer; it helps to cool down the body a bit on really hot days. Culinary traditions in warm climates all over the world pair cilantro and lime. Topping your food with fresh lime and cilantro is one of the best things you can do for your belly: it cools you down, disinfects your food and supports optimal digestion of nutrients.

Like other carminative herbs, cilantro can relax sphincters in the digestive tract and help to expel uncomfortable gas, making it the perfect fresh garnish for beans and bean soups. When you want to put it into soups, just add fresh cilantro right before serving.

**PROJECTS:** herbal water, herbal drinks, herbal smoothies, herbal vinegar, herbal oil, herbal pesto

---

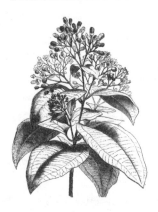

**COMMON NAME: cinnamon**

**BOTANICAL NAME: *Cinnamomum zeylanicum***

**PART USED: dried inner bark**

**GARDENING TIPS:** Cinnamon is cultivated in tropical forests in Indonesia and other parts of Asia.

**PROPERTIES:** alterative, anthelmintic, antibacterial, anticatarrh, antifungal, anti-inflammatory, antispasmodic, antiviral, astringent, expectorant, hemostat

**USES:** Cinnamon is one of those herbs that many hands play a part in growing and harvesting, yet it arrives wrapped in plastic and packed into cardboard boxes without my knowing who really did what to get it to me. We are so fortunate to have access to such a fanciful selection of herbs; they come in from all over the world to heighten the taste and aroma in our lives. From faraway island shores and deep forested jungles, the destination is my doorstep. We take it for granted, but it really is an incredible gift to have access to the earth's healing pharmacy as we do.

Cinnamon is one of the first herbs that I used as a child. My recollection of using spices is limited, but I remember adding cinnamon to pies and cobblers and putting it on white bread toast with sugar. I ditched the sugar and evolved into eating whole-grain sprouted breads sprinkled with a mixture of cardamom and cinnamon.

Put this energizing herb in a shaker and keep it on the table. When he was three years old, my son started shaking cinnamon on his oatmeal and creamed rice. It aids in digesting desserts, smoothies, and meals that contain grains and cold dairy such as milk, yogurt, and ice cream. Cinnamon increases warmth and circulation and supports efficient digestion of fats and cold foods. Cinnamon helps counteract the congestion that can accompany dairy foods.

We know cinnamon is one of the main spices for desserts, but we don't usually think of it as a woman's herb. You will be pleased with what a few cups of tea made from this sweet and spicy brown bark can do for menstrual cramps. It relaxes the uterine muscle and calms painful uterine spasms. Many women have expressed their astonishment at how effective cinnamon is for calming their menstrual pain. Menstrual discomfort suffered for years is suddenly appeased with some tea that looks like mud.

Cinnamon-ginger tea is a time-tested remedy for the onset of colds. If you are suffering with a cough, cold, or sore throat, consider using cinnamon to quicken your healing process. Cinnamon will dissolve mucus and help resolve irritating coughs and bronchial congestion. It is a natural cure for allergic rhinitis and clears stagnation throughout the respiratory tract. Cinnamon tea also makes an effective mouthwash for gum inflammation.

**PROJECTS:** herbal water, herbal drinks, herbal smoothies, herbal honey, herbal cordial, herbal oil, herbal ghee, herbal sprinkle, herbal bath and foot soak

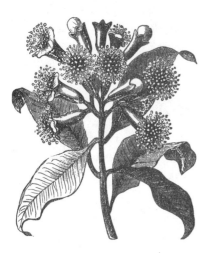

**COMMON NAME:** clove

**BOTANICAL NAME:** *Eugenia caryophyllata*

**PART USED:** dried flower bud

**GARDENING TIPS:** Clove is a tropical plant requiring warm and humid growing conditions.

**PROPERTIES:** analgesic, anesthetic, anthelmintic, antibacterial, antifungal, anti-inflammatory, antioxidant, antispasmodic, antiviral, carminative, expectorant, nutritive

**USES:** Once you realize the immensity of this spice's healing capacity, you will seek out more ways to use it in your food preparation. Fortunately, that isn't too difficult; the rich, warm taste and aroma of this spice has people wanting to hang around the kitchen. Realtors put candles and aromatherapy products scented with clove, cinnamon, and orange in houses they want to sell. The scent of cloves elicits homey feelings of satisfaction and contentment.

This richly pungent and energizing dried flower bud has been used in healing acne, colds, constipation, coughs, dyspepsia, indigestion, intestinal parasites, muscle spasms, nausea, skin ulcers, sores, and toothaches. You can suck on it when you have a toothache, cook it into applesauce, or sprinkle it in your coffee. Cloves provide a pleasant accent to sweet and savory dishes and punctuate the flavor of cookies/biscuits and pies.

It is a good thing we use cloves in pudding and pies, because cloves are an antidote to the mucus-forming nature of desserts. Heavy desserts are known to clog the sinuses, dull the mind, and produce phlegm. Cloves open the sinuses, encourage mental clarity, and resolve phlegm.

Cloves are also highly antibacterial, helping rid the body of undesirable microorganisms. At the onset of a cold, drink a tea made with black pepper–clove honey or drink elderberry, cardamom, and clove cordial after dinner.

Cloves expel the bacteria-infected mucus that can instigate sinus problems or leave one susceptible to coughs and bronchial infections.

**PROJECTS:** herbal water, herbal drinks, herbal smoothies, herbal honey, herbal vinegar, herbal cordials, herbal oil, herbal ghee, herbal sprinkle, herbal bath and foot soak

---

**COMMON NAME: coriander**

**BOTANICAL NAME:** *Coriandrum sativum*

**PART USED: seed**

**GARDENING TIPS:** Coriander is the seed of the same plant that gives us cilantro. It likes a moist place in the center of the garden with partial shade. It does not tolerate frost or high temperatures.

**PROPERTIES:** antibacterial, anti-inflammatory, antifungal, antioxidant, antispasmodic, carminative, diuretic, nervine

**USES:** Coriander relieves intestinal cramps and spasms, helps with anxiety and nervous tension, and can help regulate an overheated digestive system. Its affinity for both the digestive and nervous system make it the people's herb, tending to everyday common ailments. Its ability to amalgamate spices into a unified blend of flavor makes it the cook's companion in the daily quest for the ultimate palate-pleasing dinner.

Coriander has a synergistic effect in spice mixtures. Its lemony taste synthesizes diverse flavors; when mixing it with other herbs you can't really go wrong. It mingles well with hot herbs like chile and mustard and also fits right in with sweet spices like cinnamon and cardamom. It is well known as a pickling spice, and it complements mustard, chutney, sauerkraut, and fermented vegetables. Coriander is abundant in spice mixtures from all over the world and holds a prominent place in many cultures' cuisines. Once hoarded by Egyptian kings and taken to the tomb by pharaohs, coriander now holds a distinguished place in my squash soup and stew blends.

Coriander is yet another herb that is superb in helping with all things digestive. When we understand that many diseases are rooted in digestive problems, then the attributes of this golden-brown seed take on more significance. Fortifying digestion is the number one way to reduce inflammatory complaints in the body such as leaky gut syndrome, allergies, and arthritis. Insufficient digestion results in a chronic inflammatory process that robs nutrients from other parts of the body, eventually exhausting the nervous system. This inflammatory cascade gobbles up potassium, depleting the nervous system and disrupting the body's chemical balance. Anxiety and nervousness follow hot on the heels of inflammation and nervous system depletion. Coriander has an anti-inflammatory effect throughout the body and is rich in potassium and other nutrients that inflammation pilfers from healthy tissue.

With such an affinity for the body and so many types of food, it is no wonder that coriander is called for in recipes almost as much as salt. I use coriander in the majority of spice combinations. Coriander and cumin are my favorite mixture for lentil soup and eggplant/aubergine dishes. In chapter 9, on herbal oils, there is a recipe for Vibrant Life Oil (page 215), which contains coriander, paprika, and clove. It is *so* delicious. Sauté your soup base vegetables in it or put it on corn on the cob! Coriander ghee is also a wonderful condiment to cook with, or add a dollop to soup just before serving. Make a coriander-cumin-fennel sprinkle and keep it on the table to spice up most grain dishes.

**PROJECTS:** herbal drinks, herbal smoothies, herbal honey, herbal vinegar, herbal cordial, herbal oil, herbal ghee, herbal pesto, herbal sprinkle, herbal bath and foot soak

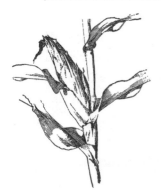

**COMMON NAME: corn silk**
**BOTANICAL NAME: *Zea mays***
**PART USED: silk**
**GARDENING TIPS:** Corn likes the full summer sunshine and lots and lots of water. It doesn't like frost, so plant it once all chances of frost have passed.

**PROPERTIES:** anti-inflammatory, astringent, cholagogue, demulcent, diuretic, nutritive

**USES:** I love corn season, as it usually means more time with friends, barbecues, and warm summer nights. When you shuck the corn for your next summer evening meal, save the corn silk! Fresh corn silk is a food that contains easily assimilated nutrients. You can brew tea with the fresh corn silk or use it as a topping for just about any salad type dish. Just make sure you mince it into tiny pieces: if you try to eat it in long strings, it will be nothing but irritating!

If you go through as much corn as we do, there is no way to eat or drink all the fresh silk, so you can dry it for later use. Pull the silk from the cob and separate it from the husk. Make sure to also save the silk that is at the top of the husk on the outside of the corn. Run your fingers through the silk a little to loosen it from being in one big clump. Place the corn silk on a flat basket and set it out on the counter to dry. Depending on the weather, this can take a few days. Once all the water is gone from the silk and it feels slightly crispy, you can store it in a jar or paper bag. Corn silk keeps this way for about one year.

Dried corn silk makes a very nice-tasting tea that is traditionally employed as an anti-inflammatory for the urinary tract. Two cups a day for several weeks helps with cystitis, urethritis, and prostatitis. It is tonic to the prostate and urinary tract and is a safe herbal tea for people of all ages. Corn silk soothes and relaxes the lining of the urinary tract and bladder, relieving irritation and improving urine flow and elimination. This is a great remedy for people with incontinence and any type of urinary discomfort. If you are prone to urinary tract infections, corn silk is the herb for you. You don't have to be inflamed to enjoy a cup of corn silk tea though. It is a demulcent, nutritive herb containing many beneficial minerals. Corn silk has a mildly sweet flavor and makes a good-tasting and refreshing summer tea for everybody. So next time you make corn on the cob, make some corn silk tea to drink after dinner.

**PROJECTS:** herbal drinks

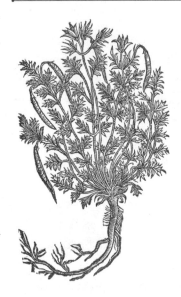

**COMMON NAME: cumin**

**BOTANICAL NAME: *Cuminum cyminum***

**PART USED: seed**

**GARDENING TIPS:** Cumin is a frost-sensitive plant that doesn't like cold climates in general. So if you live in an area with mild winters, try growing cumin in porous soil and dappled light.

**PROPERTIES:** anthelmintic, antibacterial, antispasmodic, carminative, emmenagogue, galactagogue, nervine

**USES:** Cumin eases coughs, supports digestion, helps with anxiety and insomnia, and contains nutritive vitamins and minerals. A little bit of cumin in spice blends adds a robust spike of flavor. Cumin is indeed one of the most versatile spices, finding itself in food everywhere. It is an ingredient in Mexican mole and Middle Eastern spice pastes. Cumin graces curry blends from various regions of the world, Italian sauce mixtures, African stews, Northern European specialty breads, meat-preserving condiments from Greece, and Asian fish sauces.

If you travel to any of these regions, indulge in all the cumin-rich sauces to protect against the ravage of rot gut that often accompanies international travel. As an anthelmintic herb, cumin helps to keep pathogens in check in the digestive tract. Carry cumin with you when you travel to faraway places or to the campground.

Cumin is also the mother's helper as it quells nausea and encourages lactation. Cumin is a staple ingredient in colic water recipes and can be used to support the healthy flow of breast milk in nursing mothers. Make a colic tea of equal parts cumin and fennel and feed it to mom and baby. It quiets the mind along with the stomach and promotes relaxation and mental clarity.

This tiny little brown seed also remedies the effects of spicy food on the stomach. Often spice mixes that have lots of hot chile will include coriander and cumin to assuage the indigestion and heartburn that can flare up after eating excessively spicy food. One of my favorite seasoning blends is cumin, coriander, and fennel. Experiment with your own three-seed ghee using cumin, celery seed, and fennel. It is the best ghee to use for scrambling eggs and sautéing onions for soup and sauce bases, or just spread it on toasted bread.

**PROJECTS:** herbal honey, herbal vinegar, herbal cordials, herbal oil, herbal ghee, herbal sprinkle, herbal bath and foot soak

---

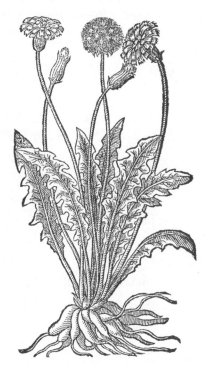

**COMMON NAME:** **dandelion leaf**

**BOTANICAL NAME:** *Taraxacum officinale*

**PART USED:** **leaf**

**GARDENING TIPS:** As far as gardening goes, dandelion loves lawns and parks and thrives in moist or dried, disturbed soil. All you have to do is restrain yourself from pulling it up when you are blessed with it growing in your yard.

**PROPERTIES:** alterative, aperient, bitter tonic, cholagogue, diuretic, galactagogue, nutritive, tonic

**USES:** I see people pulling up dandelion, cursing it, kicking it, and spraying chemicals all around it. What people don't know is that this jagged-edged green weed that causes them so much trouble is a powerhouse healing herb full of worthy nutrients. Most everyone could prosper from the high content of vitamins A, C, and E that this herb imparts. Dandelion is free, grows without care, and then we pull it up and poison it—what an interesting paradox. What we need is right in front of us, yet we go to extended trouble to eradicate it. This gives us a glimpse into our sometimes upside-down relationship with nature.

The applications for this plant go on and on. Its nutritive qualities alone are reason enough to absorb it into your diet. Dandelion leaf is a mineral-rich bitter tonic that is one of the best herbs to munch on in spring salads. I put it into my salad and salad dressing. Try making a fresh dandelion leaf vinegar and dressing foods with this liquid multivitamin garnish.

Dandelion leaf is bitter, which is a flavor that we need more of in our diet. The common menu is laden with sugar and low-quality salt. Sweet and salty are the tastes that most people crave. If bitters are new territory, it can take a little getting used to. Once you take up residence with bitter foods, you notice how much more robust your digestion is, and you will develop a hankering for a bitter aperitif before dinner.

The bitter taste of dandelion leaf increases the flow of saliva, which contains antibacterial substances and enzymes that commence the breakdown of your food. Dandelion leaf also stimulates digestive secretions throughout the digestive tract. Dandelion leaves enhance the strength of peristalsis and stimulate the flow of stomach secretions and other helpful digestive substances. The salivation that is stimulated by bitter herbs is an invaluable aspect of nutrient assimilation. This initial digesting and disinfection is done in the mouth so the rest of the digestive tract doesn't have to compensate for what could have taken place in the mouth. It isn't something that makes a difference in one day, but over time, a lifestyle of taking bitter, saliva-activating herbs means better health.

Dandelion greens are tonic to the liver and kidneys. They help resolve fluid congestion and are one of the most nutrient-dense greens that nature has to offer. Make a bitter cordial with dandelion leaf, mugwort leaf, and a little ginger to sip before a meal, or splash your steamed vegetables with minced dandelion leaves to rouse the digestion of a lion.

**PROJECTS:** herbal drinks, herbal smoothies, herbal vinegar, herbal pesto, herbal sprinkle

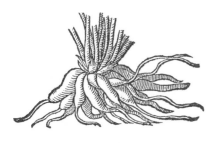

**COMMON NAME:** dandelion root

**BOTANICAL NAME:** *Taraxacum officinale*

**PART USED: root**

**GARDENING TIPS:** See dandelion leaf, page 73.

**PROPERTIES:** alterative, antibacterial, anti-inflammatory, aperient, bitter tonic, cholagogue, diuretic, galactagogue, nutritive, tonic

**USES:** Dandelion root is a nutritive tonic that enhances overall wellness. Its generous content of minerals and electrolytes categorizes this herb as a general health-promoting tonic herb. The next time you weed your yard, dig up a dandelion root, wash it, chop it, and add the fresh root to your soups, tea, or a detoxification bath. It can be consumed fresh, or you can dry it for later use.

Dandelion helps facilitate optimum digestion in many ways. The bitter taste of dandelion root stimulates receptor sites on the tongue that send information to the digestive tract. The bitter flavor message initiates gastric secretions from the stomach, liver, and pancreas. Gastric secretions naturally wane with age. Assimilating bitter foods into the diet in small amounts helps maintain healthy digestive function and premium nutrient absorption into the later years of life. Dandelion root contains inulin, which nourishes the beneficial bacteria in the gastrointestinal tract and enhances digestion. Healthful beneficial bacteria play a significant role in how well you assimilate what you eat and therefore your energy and vitality. Check out the recipe for Dandelion Mocha on page 143. It is a great pick-me-up that goes easy on the liver.

This simple root also supports healthy liver and gallbladder function. It stimulates the flow of bile, which breaks down cholesterol and fat. Dandelion nurtures the liver in its assimilation and storage of vitamins, minerals, and sugars. It improves blood filtration to remove old cells and harmful bacteria and helps maintain a healthy hormone balance. Liver health also plays an important role in regulating blood sugar and excreting accumulated waste. We are endowed with a liver that performs a thousand functions. It is just plain courteous to eat some herbs to reciprocate all the liver does to make us happy.

Dandelion root is a popular spring tonic used to help shed the sluggishness of winter. It is also a gentle diuretic that moderates premenstrual fluid retention. The root is a useful remedy for urinary tract irritation and has an overall restorative effect on the urinary tract. No wonder dandelion root is considered a cure-all. From the lawn to your liver, put this curative root where it belongs: in the cupboard.

Do not use dandelion root with bile duct or gallbladder disease.

**PROJECTS:** herbal honey, herbal vinegar, herbal cordial, herbal sprinkle, herbal bath and foot soak

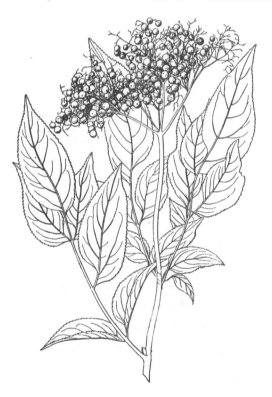

**COMMON NAME: elderberry**

**BOTANICAL NAME:** *Sambucus mexicana and nigra* (blue and black elderberry varieties only; red elderberries are not edible.)

**PART USED: berry**

**GARDENING TIPS:** Whenever you see elder, you know there is water nearby, as it likes to keep its roots wet. Elderberry grows well in the sun with a bit of shade. It grows along the riverbanks where I live in the Sacramento Valley. It loves to be well watered but can survive sweltering summer days when the rivers run dry. Once established, it hangs on through intense drought and heat and always comes back in the spring.

**PROPERTIES:** alterative, anti-inflammatory, antioxidant, antiviral, aperient, expectorant, nutritive

**USES:** Elderberry cordial is first on the list to subdue cold and flu symptoms. I can't even tell you how many colds have started and then not progressed due to the aid of elderberry cordial. Put elderberry honey on pancakes or drink a shot of elderberry cordial before bed. Elderberry enhances the immune system, and its antiviral properties inhibit flu virus from penetrating cell membranes. Elderberry tea, cordial, or honey can be used to prevent respiratory viral infections.

Elderberry remedies work best for you if taken at the very onset of symptoms, before the virus takes hold. When someone says, "I woke up with a sore throat," the symptoms are pretty obvious by that point. There were probably a few signs of susceptibility in the days preceding waking up with the sore throat. It is important to develop an awareness of presickness symptoms. These are the more subtle changes that you experience before the coughs and sneezes and before your symptoms become acute. It is the awareness of these subacute warning signals that give you a jump on beating a cold. With this consciousness, you can begin using elderberries when they work most efficiently, at the very onset of cold symptoms. Don't wait until you know you are sick. At the first sign of a tickle in the throat, a drop in energy, burning eyes, achy muscles, or any other preflu symptoms, think of elderberry.

These highly medicinal bluish-black berries are rich in vitamins A and C and are loaded with flavonoids that are tonic to the cardiovascular system. Elderberries also have a long history of being used to pacify rheumatic pain. If you can feel the weather in your joints long before it starts raining, elderberry is a good herb to invite into the pantry. Make a cordial with elderberry and a little cinnamon and nutmeg and have a sip in the evening after dinner. I make lots of elderberry cordial every year, and there is always someone who needs it.

Fresh elderberries are best made into vinegar, cordial, and other foods and medicines. If you eat too many fresh elderberries, they can give you a stomachache.

**PROJECTS:** herbal drinks, herbal vinegar, herbal cordial

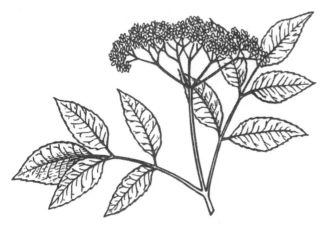

**COMMON NAME:** elder
flower
**BOTANICAL NAME:**
*Sambucus mexicana and nigra*
**PART USED:** flower
**GARDENING TIPS:**
See elderberry, page 76
**PROPERTIES:** alterative, anti-catarrhal, anti-inflammatory, demulcent, expectorant, vulnerary
**USES:** I keep a file on all the plants that I have studied over the years. Elder flower is one of the plants of my childhood, and for almost twenty-five years, I have been gathering pages and pages of notes on this lacey yellow flower. I write down remedies, recipes, rumors, poetry about plants, success stories, scientific studies, and other ditties. In my notes for elder flower it says, "Drink elder flower tea for a dozen miseries."

Elder flowers are a cooling decongestant for the respiratory mucosa. They are the perfect herb with which to make summer drinks. We celebrate summertime with elder flower fizzes and elder flower lemonade. It keeps us cool while holding summer allergies at bay. Rich in quercetin, elder flowers are noted for their anti-inflammatory effects on hay fever symptoms. Quercetin is shown to have cancer-reducing activity and alleviates hay fever and sinusitis.

In the winter, we drink hot elder flower tea at the very first sign of a cold that starts with a runny nose. Elder flowers help with allergies, earache, rhinitis, sinusitis, and all mucus problems of the upper respiratory tract. It is an anticatarrhal herb, helping to moderate excess mucus. When the front of your face feels as if it is dripping from your head along with the snot, think of using elder flower. Elder flowers are legendary in their ability to arrest nasal discharge and drainage.

The entire digestive tract is protected by the lubrication of mucus. Some mucus is good, but too much mucus is not so good. There is a balance of mucus that is beneficial and healthful; when there is excess mucus, it means something is out of whack. It is important to identify the source of the excess mucus. Often food allergies and digestive distress are at the root of the problem. Identifying food allergies, using anticatarrhal herbs, and supporting optimum digestion can help relieve the overproduction of mucus. But when we are stuck with an exorbitant amount of fluid dripping and draining from various locations, it is time to engage the snot-busting features of elder flower.

This sweetly fragrant flower also soothes the skin. Elder flowers clear heat from the skin, heal bruises and burns, and help reduce swelling. They make an exceptional face wash, softening the skin and clearing the complexion. Elder flower–rose petal vinegar is a great topical remedy for sunburns, and I hope that you take time to enjoy the luxury of an elder flower and lavender bath.

**PROJECTS:** herbal water, herbal drinks, herbal smoothies, herbal honey, herbal vinegar, herbal cordial, herbal oils, herbal bath and foot soak

---

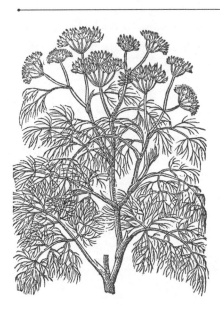

**COMMON NAME: fennel seed**

**BOTANICAL NAME: *Foeniculum vulgare***

**PART USED: seed**

**GARDENING TIPS:** We have renamed fennel the highway plant. It grows wild all along the sides of the highway in central California. The more disturbed the area, the more it grows. It likes any kind of soil and lots of sun and can grow without much water. The problem with fennel is that each year it throws off thousands of seeds and can colonize your garden.

You can eat the root, leaves, and flowers of this plant, but recipes in this book refer to the seeds that are harvested in the late summer.

**PROPERTIES:** anthelmintic, antibacterial, anti-inflammatory, antispasmodic, carminative, demulcent, expectorant, galactagogue, nervine, tonic

**USES:** Fennel has always grown in abundance where I live, and it just gives and gives. I love this herb. Maybe I say that about a lot of plants, but I really do love using fennel seed in my everyday life. How do people live without it? Especially if you have children, get some fennel seed and begin harnessing its medicinal virtues. Fennel is one of the best herbs for settling a nervous, upset stomach. Children usually enjoy the licorice-like flavor, and it helps them with stomachaches, constipation, coughs, and excess mucus. If you are a nursing mom, drink fennel tea to soothe your baby's colic. Fennel is the primary ingredient in the old gripe water remedy for colic. Steep fennel seeds, chamomile, and ginger in apple cider vinegar to make your own gripe water for comforting digestive complaints.

Fennel seed is a reliable antispasmodic and is one of the best remedies for abdominal cramping associated with poor digestion. Its aromatic, carminative properties help with nausea, belching, and bloating caused by indigestion. Fennel seed improves vision, enhances mental clarity, and has an overall restorative and calming effect. Warm fennel tea is comfort in a cup. It just settles everything the way it is supposed to be. Maybe you don't know what you need; let fennel take care of it.

Fennel is a staple ingredient in the food, drink, and herbal condiments in our house. It has a delicious flavor and aroma that most people enjoy. Drink fennel seed tea in the winter or chew on fennel seeds to help digest heavy meals. Fennel seed tea can also stop a chronic cough, fennel seed water complements any seafood dish, and fennel honey livens up an afternoon tea.

**PROJECTS:** herbal water, herbal drinks, herbal smoothies, herbal honey, herbal vinegar, herbal cordial, herbal oil, herbal ghee, herbal pesto, herbal sprinkle, herbal bath and foot soak

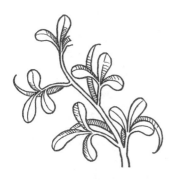

**COMMON NAME:** **fenugreek**

**BOTANICAL NAME:** *Trigonella foenumgraecum*

**PART USED:** **seed**

**GARDENING TIPS:** After the frost is over, plant this legume/pulse in the spring once the weather has warmed up in full sun. Grow it as you would any bean plant, in full sun with rich, fertile, well-drained soil. Fenugreek makes a good cover crop for fixing nitrogen in the soil. Keep it well watered throughout the summer and let it go to seed to harvest for food and medicine.

**PROPERTIES:** Antibacterial, anticatarrh, anti-inflammatory, antioxidant, aperient, bitter tonic, carminative, circulatory stimulant, demulcent, emmenagogue, expectorant, galactagogue, nervine, nutritive, tonic, vulnerary

**USES:** My first encounter with fenugreek was a rumor espousing its notability as an effective deodorant. I didn't really believe it, but I tried it anyway. I drank fenugreek seed tea for several days, and much to my surprise, my underarm sweat started to exude a sweet, candylike smell. If you don't like the smell of your sweat, trade your deodorant out for fenugreek. It really does give you sweet sweat.

Fenugreek is a favorite sprouted seed to put on salads. Just soak them in water overnight, put them in a sprouting jar, and watch your indoor garden grow. The packed-in nutrients that are released to feed the seed now can feed your body. We eat these sprouts all summer long. Growing them takes little effort, and you can mix them into just about any type of lunch. The festive yellow sprouted seed has a signature maple syrup scent and is a powerhouse of vitamins and minerals.

Fenugreek is a nourishing tonic. Its rich makeup of nutrients revitalizes and restores the body. It also helps to regulate blood sugar and is well known for its ability to bring on delayed menstruation. Fenugreek is a galactagogue and has a reputation of increasing the flow of breast milk in breast-feeding women and in farm animals. Fenugreek and fennel tea is the nursing moms' panacea.

Dried fenugreek seed is as hard as a little stone, but once it is soaked in water for a few hours, it turns into a gooey slimeball. Slippery slime is actually good for us. This demulcent quality soothes and heals our mucous membrane, which we have a lot of: our external mucous membrane—our skin—covers us from head to toe, and our internal mucous membrane is the skin that covers us from mouth to anus. That is a lot of surface area for fenugreek to work on. The mucilaginous quality of fenugreek reduces inflammation of all the mucous membrane. It helps with inflammation in the sinus, mouth, throat, lungs, and colon. Sinusitis, gastritis, irritable bowel syndrome, coughs, sore throats, and hemorrhoids are common inflammatory complaints that fenugreek can help pacify. Fenugreek tea is a good skin wash for topical inflammation including minor cuts, scrapes, and bug bites. If you suffer with irritated and itchy skin, try taking fenugreek baths.

Fenugreek is impossible to powder with home equipment, so either buy it powdered or soak the whole seed overnight in a little water and then mash it with olive oil to make a spice paste. Pack fenugreek paste on fish before baking or use it to cover any red, itchy, inflamed patch of skin on your body. Powdered fenugreek can be added to baking flour for pancakes and savory muffins or put into a tea for a sore throat gargle.

**PROJECTS:** herbal drinks, herbal honey, herbal vinegar, herbal cordial, herbal oils, herbal ghee, herbal sprinkle, herbal bath and foot soak

---

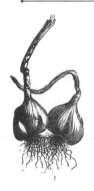

**COMMON NAME: garlic**
**BOTANICAL NAME: *Allium sativum***
**PART USED: bulb**
**GARDENING TIPS:** Garlic likes lots of well-drained, fluffy, fertile soil. Plant it in the fall in the sunniest spot you can find and dig it up in midsummer.

**PROPERTIES:** anthelmintic, antibacterial, antifungal, antioxidant, antispasmodic, carminative, expectorant

**USES:** So many of our foods are endowed with highly medicinal properties, but a lot of that knowledge has fallen out of household awareness. Not so with garlic. It is one of the foods that most everyone still remembers to take to deter colds and flu. Maybe it is the pungent smell that won't let us forget its power. When you put thyme in the spaghetti sauce, you don't really think of it as a curative ingredient, but with garlic, there is a medicinal memory. Once you chop it open, you know you are working with a potent remedy. Offending your family with constant garlic breath must have some kind of payoff.

In Ayurvedic medicine, garlic is called the slayer of monsters. Odysseus used garlic wine to save himself from the spells of the sorceresses. The Romans carried garlic into war for protection. Battling the ills of modern society, it is the number one selling herb in Germany and the second most popular herbal supplement in the United States. Current studies document that garlic lives up to its age-old lore of providing healing and protection on many different levels.

Garlic has been clinically studied as a heart medicine for more than thirty years, and its usefulness in supporting people with hypertension and diabetes is well documented. Garlic prevents blood clots and protects arteries from age-related stiffening. It lowers high blood pressure and reduces the risk of stroke. With cardiovascular disease being a major cause of death in the United States, pass the garlic press please.

Garlic contains several sulfur compounds that are antimicrobial. Garlic boosts the production of white blood cells, helping to fight off bacteria, parasites, and viruses. It is effective against many antibiotic-resistant strains of bacteria. If you are getting sick, eat garlic. The antimicrobial properties of garlic are more effective if the garlic is eaten fresh. You may not feel like eating fresh raw garlic, and for some people it causes digestive upset. Adding minced fresh garlic to food or putting it on bread with butter is a good way to help it go down easier. If I feel like I have been exposed to a cold or just feel a little run-down, I keep the garlic press at the table and just press out minced fresh garlic onto whatever I am eating for dinner.

Fresh garlic can trigger gastrointestinal disturbance in some people. If fresh garlic irritates your stomach, make Tamari Honey Marinade (page 169), let it age for several months, and watch how you can eat garlic as if it were candy! You can also halve a clove and rub it on the bottom of your feet. The antibacterial oils enter the bloodstream through the feet and help fight off a cold without you even having to eat the garlic! Watch out, garlic foot rubs causes garlic breath!

**PROJECTS:** herbal honey, herbal vinegar, herbal cordial, herbal oils, herbal ghee, herbal pesto, herbal sprinkle, herbal foot soak

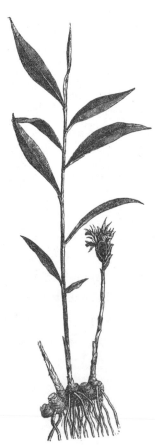

**COMMON NAME: ginger**

**BOTANICAL NAME:** *Zingiber officinale*

**PART USED: root**

**GARDENING TIPS:** Cultivated in tropical regions, ginger thrives in hot and damp environments.

**PROPERTIES:** antibacterial, antifungal, anti-inflammatory, antioxidant, antiviral, carminative, circulatory stimulant, expectorant, rubefacient

**USES:** Ginger helps with colds, flu, and coughs. It relieves nausea, motion sickness, seasickness, and sore throats. Ginger increases circulation, gets rid of mucus congestion, settles an upset stomach, dispels gas, relieves aches and pains, reduces inflammation and menstrual cramps, supports the pancreas, and stimulates digestion. (Let me catch my breath; shall I go on?) Ginger root is truly the universal medicine. Its warmth fills our tea, honey, and cordials all winter long. Any time you have some mucus sneaking up on you, use a ginger sprinkle on your morning foods or make a ginger–star anise honey and take it by the teaspoonful. The ginger will cause you to perspire and sweat out the cold.

I really could just fill the rest of the pages in this book with why ginger is one of the most amazing substances on the planet, but I want room to share all of my recipes with you, so let's just talk about a few things in regard to ginger. To begin with, fresh ginger contains a proteolytic enzyme that reduces inflammation and helps to regenerate and repair damaged tissue including scar tissue. If you have inflammation that causes you aches and pains, use ginger. If you have arthritis, make friends with ginger. Drink it as an after-dinner tea, grate it fresh into your salad, and take ginger-rosemary baths.

Inflammatory conditions plague many women during menstruation. You can find relief from PMS symptoms by using ginger. Ginger inhibits inflammatory prostaglandins that contribute to menstrual cramps and other PMS symptoms. Incorporate ginger tea and foot soaks into your personal care rituals to support menstruation.

Diabetes is becoming more prevalent in the health care concerns of people of all ages. If you are worried about diabetes, add ginger to your soups and salads to enhance pancreatic function. Ginger demonstrates significant efficacy in lowering the blood levels of triglycerides that are common in diabetes. Anything that raises your blood sugar levels can increase your triglycerides. Elevated triglycerides are indicated in diabetes, heart disease, and risk of stroke. Reduce your sugar intake and include ginger in your daily meals to reduce triglyceride levels and support your pancreas.

Many people rely on ginger for preventing nausea, motion sickness, and seasickness. Clinical trials show that ginger rivals nausea drugs for chemotherapy-induced nausea. With so many healing benefits, experiment with how you like to use ginger in your culinary escapades. I love starting cold days off with a cup of ginger-honey tea. It moves my blood, activates my brain, and provides protection against who knows what.

**PROJECTS:** herbal water, herbal drinks, herbal smoothies, herbal honey, herbal vinegar, herbal cordial, herbal oil, herbal ghee, herbal pesto, herbal sprinkle, herbal bath and foot soak

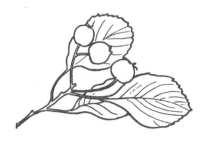

**COMMON NAME:** **hawthorn berry**

**BOTANICAL NAME:** *Cratageus spp.*

**PART USED:** **berry**

**GARDENING TIPS:** Finally, after ten years, my hawthorn tree gave me the first harvest of berries. I thought that it took too long, but when I remembered that these beautiful trees live to be more than two hundred years old, I realized that ten years just seemed like a long time to me and not to the tree. Hawthorn is a very adaptive tree. I grew it in the Sacramento Valley in full sun with limited water. It will also thrive in cold weather and icy winters. There are hundreds of varieties of hawthorn trees that have adjusted to a wide variety of weather conditions.

**PROPERTIES:** adaptogen, anti-inflammatory, antioxidant, antispasmodic, astringent, bitter tonic, emmenagogue, tonic

**USES:** Hawthorn berry is one of our best herbal tonics for the heart. It is a little red berry that is easily added to food. Combine hawthorn berry, cinnamon, and rose hips into a sprinkle for breakfast foods and smoothies. Feed your heart with hawthorn berry–cinnamon tea or make a hawthorn berry, dandelion root, and ginger cordial for an after-meal treat. I add hawthorn berry, lavender, and lemon balm honey to desserts and use it to sweeten drinks. Put a dash of powdered hawthorn berry in any smoothie or make a hawthorn honey to sweeten specialty drinks. Try some of my recipes or find your own way to include this delicious heart food in your cookery.

The well-substantiated uses of hawthorn berry include lowering blood pressure, improving circulatory disorders, and enhancing cardiac output. Hawthorn strengthens the heart and promotes longevity. It has numerous positive effects on cardiac function and is considered a tonic for the circulatory system. Hawthorn helps to maintain healthy veins, arteries, and capillaries. It decreases capillary permeability and fragility and supports the flow of blood to the heart.

With cardiovascular disease being such a major health concern, isn't it great to have an herb that has a beneficial and restorative effect on the entire cardiovascular system? Add some hawthorn berry and rose petal honey to a cup of hot water, relax, and let nature help you with your health.

Saturated with flavonoids, hawthorn berry helps to stabilize collagen and prevent collagen tissue loss caused by inflammation and oxidation. Collagen is the protein that helps make up blood vessels and is responsible for maintaining the integrity of tendons, ligaments, and cartilage. Collagen is also the main protein in skin. When it is healthy, skin is glowing and resilient. The rich red hawthorn berry supports healthy collagen and connective tissue throughout the body.

Hawthorn berry contains rutin, which enhances vitamin C activity and strengthens capillaries for people who bruise a lot. Do you know someone who looks as if they have been in a wrestling match every time they bump into something? Make them a hawthorn berry–rose hip ghee.

Hawthorn berries can be contra-indicated while taking cardiac medications.

**PROJECTS:** herbal drinks, herbal smoothies, herbal honey, herbal vinegar, herbal cordial, herbal ghee, herbal sprinkle, herbal bath and foot soak

---

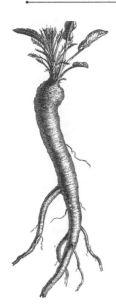

**COMMON NAME: horseradish**

**BOTANICAL NAME:** *Armoracia rusticana*

**PART USED: root**

**GARDENING TIPS:** I have grown this herb for years. I completely ignore what kind of soil it has or how much water it gets. It dies back every winter and in the spring comes back almost twice the size it was the previous year. I harvest roots from it several times a year, and it just keeps getting bigger and bigger. It isn't sensitive to cold environments and thrives with very little care.

**PROPERTIES:** anthelmintic, antibacterial, anticatarrhal, antioxidant, aperient, carminative, diuretic, expectorant, rubefacient

**USES:** Have you ever eaten too much horseradish sauce and felt as if the top of your head were going to blow off? Eyes turning red, tears gushing down your face, ears tingling, snot dripping from your nose—and then suddenly, it all stops. You catch your breath and notice your head is clear, your sinuses have opened up, and you feel pretty good! This experience gives some insight into the medicinal activity of this hot, spicy, pungent root.

If you deal with chronic sinus congestion, get out the sinus-plunging herb. Make some horseradish root vinegar, or check out the recipe for Fire Cider on page 178. Take 1 teaspoon of the Fire Cider (5 ml) a couple of times a day. For many years, we lived in a beautiful canyon that was a bit too shady for me in the winter. The dampness and darkness slowed down my metabolism, and every winter I had to take special care of my sinuses. Horseradish vinegar was a primary remedy for keeping my sinusitis from progressing into an infection.

As you have probably already discovered, horseradish increases metabolism and circulation, dissolves accumulated mucus, clears the sinus, warms the body, and drains any mucus that might be hiding. Excess mucus is a breeding ground for colds and bacteria that can cause infections. So moving it out, even if it means lots of spouting snot, is good. It is the stuck mucus that provides a medium for bacteria to take hold in the sinuses. Keeping the nasal passages clear of mucus helps prevent sinusitis and sinus infections. Think of horseradish as Drano for the head.

Horseradish is best used when grated fresh. You can keep a fresh root in your fridge for up to two months. I dig up a little root from my garden every few months and keep it in the refrigerator, grating it fresh into food. If you have dried horseradish root, rehydrate it with a little water for fifteen minutes before using it.

Horseradish is an intensely hot root with a spiky taste. It is meant to be used in small amounts to garnish rich food. Too much of it just overwhelms any other taste you might like to enjoy. Horseradish loses its flavor when cooked, so preserve it in condiments or add it fresh to your food. I like to sprinkle a tiny bit of horseradish root on egg salad, sandwich spreads, steamed greens, potatoes, hot quiche, and avocados. It goes well with root vegetables and rich meals containing beef, salmon, and cream. Horseradish vinegar is a secret ingredient in my potato salad.

Horseradish is high in vitamins A and C and rich in iron, calcium, magnesium, and potassium. The antioxidant properties prevent the oxidation that can harm tissues and cause premature aging. Horseradish is in the same family as broccoli and contains the same constituents that have broccoli classified as a cancer-fighting food. This hot root strengthens circulation and increases the excretion rate of toxic compounds in the body. Garnish your food with it or just chew on a small piece of root if your sinuses are bothering you.

**PROJECTS:** herbal honey, herbal vinegar, herbal cordial, herbal ghee, herbal pesto, herbal sprinkle, herbal bath and foot soak

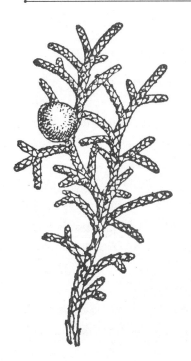

**COMMON NAME: juniper berry**

**BOTANICAL NAME:** *Juniperus communis*

**PART USED: berry**

**GARDENING TIPS:** Juniper can withstand hot, dry, poor soil and freezing winters. It is a drought-tolerant tree that will hang on in just about any condition, but don't overwater it or plant it in the shade. I have seen Juniper trees at 8,000 feet (2,440 meters) in the Sierra Nevada mountain range growing in dry, compacted soil in the blistering sun.

**PROPERTIES:** analgesic, antibacterial, anti-inflammatory, antiviral, astringent, carminative, circulatory stimulant, diuretic, expectorant

**USES:** There are a multitude of uses for juniper berries. Add them to seasonings for fish, wild meats, and fermenting vegetables. Mix a little powdered juniper berry into pancake batter, warm breakfast grains, and cookie dough. Make an invigorating juniper berry oil and use it to rub on sore muscles or to spice up your marinade. Juniper vinegar is an affective hair rinse for dandruff and can also be used as an antifungal skin wash. Juniper berries are anti-inflammatory and provide comfort for strained muscles, an achy back, and arthritic pain. Put them into your bathtub or massage juniper berry oil into stiff muscles.

All purple and blue foods contain flavonoids that are most commonly known for stimulating antioxidant activity in the body. Juniper berries contain a treasure trove of flavonoids that strengthen connective tissue in arteries and veins. They protect against allergens, carcinogens, and inflammation and have a rebuilding effect on ligaments and cartilage. Just a few berries go a long way.

As people age, they often experience cold extremities, weary eyes, and deficiency in blood circulation. Juniper is a circulatory stimulant helping the body to get to the edges of itself. Herbs that help improve circulation are beneficial allies as they increase the surface area that the blood can deliver nutrients to and eliminate waste from.

Juniper berries also have a dependable diuretic action that relieves cystitis, urethritis, premenstrual water retention, and bloating. Juniper berries are antiseptic and disinfect the urinary tract as they are excreted in the urine.

If you experience muscle stress and tension from working on the computer or driving in traffic, come home to a purifying and rejuvenating bath of juniper and rosemary. Chew on a few of the tangy, sweet, and bitter-tasting blue berries for a sore throat or to enhance circulation and lymph drainage. Enjoy the piney juniper flavor in a cold and flu prevention cordial. I love to put juniper berries in my bath and then use juniper berry oil for an after-bath body oil. This is a superb treatment for the winter doldrums. Use juniper berries in small amounts, and avoid altogether with kidney disease.

**PROJECTS:** herbal water, herbal drink, herbal smoothies, herbal honey, herbal vinegar, herbal cordial, herbal oil, herbal ghee, herbal sprinkle, herbal bath and foot soak

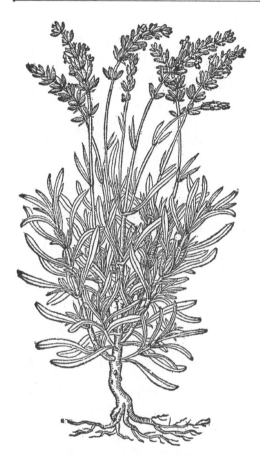

**COMMON NAME: lavender**
**BOTANICAL NAME:**
*Lavendula spp.*
**PART USED: flower and leaf**
**GARDENING TIPS:** Lavender likes to grow lavishly in the sun in well-drained soil. It does not do well in prolonged hard frost or frost immediately following extended rains. Twice in the past twenty years there has been a combination of rain and frost that killed all the lavender in our neighborhood. Lavender loves to live in a mild coastal climate placed in a sunny position. Living next to a sunny beach sounds good to me. One mistake people make with lavender is overwatering it. Lavender likes a deep watering once in a while.

**PROPERTIES:** analgesic, anti-bacterial, anticatarrhal, anti-fungal, anti-inflammatory, antispasmodic, carminative, nervine, vulnerary

**USES:** You will love the medicinal and culinary versatility of this herb. Whip up a lavender oil and then use it in your pesto, soups, stir-fries, sauces, and marinades. Let lavender permeate your meals in the form of a vinegar added to drinks, dipping sauces, and salad dressings. Rub your meats with lavender-rosemary salt and dazzle your guests with lavender lemonade. When you can't find anything else to do with it in the kitchen, put it into baths and foot soaks and pamper yourself with luxurious lavender massage oil.

Relaxation is what usually comes to mind when we think of lavender, but it has antibacterial properties as well that make it useful to cook with during cold and flu season. Lavender tea is a stress tamer and cold buster. Lavender cordial, lavender honey, and lavender vinegar all find their way into the preventative health care focus of the winter menu.

I take advantage of the antiseptic temperament of lavender and use lavender vinegar to clean my house. The root of the word "lavender" comes from the Latin word "laver," which means "to wash." Disinfect your home by boiling lavender in a large pot with the lid off the pot. The aromatic oils fill the air, sanitizing and energetically cleaning the environment.

Lavender is also an amazing topical skin healer and is helpful in easing pestilent skin conditions such as athlete's foot, rashes, eczema, and psoriasis. Take a bath to cool your skin and calm your mind. Soak yourself in the fragrance of lavender when you are mentally or physically worn out. A lavender bath also serves as a refreshing tonic that can relieve headaches, muscle strain, stress, tension, and general aches and pains. If you are prone to headaches, try taking lavender and rosemary baths on a regular basis.

Lavender really is the queen of nerve tonics. It helps you respond to the stressors of life in a less stressful way. A strengthening tonic to the nervous system, lavender helps with irritability and restlessness, calms anger and agitation, and invokes an uplifted feeling of well-being. Softening the impact of stress is a tall order these days. Herbs that heal the body and calm the mind are in high demand. "Tranquility," "serenity," "stillness," and "repose" are all words used to described the results of lavender consumption. Plant some lavender.

**PROJECTS:** herbal water, herbal drinks, herbal smoothies, herbal honey, herbal vinegar, herbal cordial, herbal oil, herbal ghee, herbal pesto, herbal sprinkle, herbal bath and foot soak

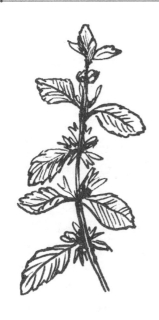

**COMMON NAME:** lemon balm

**BOTANICAL NAME:** *Melissa officinalis*

**PART USED:** leaf and flower

**GARDENING TIPS:** Lemon balm is one of those plants that push through asphalt and sidewalk cracks. It grows anywhere and likes sun or semishade. Once it sprouts in your garden, you will never get rid of it. It will attach itself to your boots and go with you when you move. If you decide you love this plant and give it good soil and water, you may end up with a field of lemon balm. "Invasive" is the description that fits the growing habits of this dear herb. I don't mind having lots of lemon balm because it keeps me happy and the bees love it.

**PROPERTIES:** antibacterial, antispasmodic, antiviral, carminative, nervine, vulnerary

**USES:** Lemon balm is another one of my favorite specialty drink herbs. Its distinctive lemon scent and pungent flavor add an evocative taste to drinks. It makes sensational lemonade and adds a nice spiking note to smoothies, and lemon balm tea can lull you to sleep. It is a fun herb to play with in cooking and concocting, but it is also seriously antiviral and an effective nerve tonic. This lemony, cooling herb hunts down viral infections and fortifies the nervous system.

Lemons balm's prestige is embedded in its usage to temper aggravated thoughts and emotions. When I first read about mood-elevating herbs, I was definitely skeptical. I could grasp wound healing and nerve calming, but could they actually elevate my mood? Without a doubt, I can attest to the consequences of drinking lemon balm: relaxation and a better mood. Lemon balm relaxes and lifts at the same time. It has a palliative effect on excessive mental activity and it moderates the intensity of mood swings and mild depression. Lemon balm is the herbal companion of choice in the face of anxiety, stress-related fatigue, and tension. It helps to resolve anxiety and emotional unrest and intervenes when emotional states take over your life. That is no small feat for a soft, light green leaf that grows like a weed.

You can jump into the stream of tradition and employ fresh lemon balm to make emotional rescue cordials. The dictionary definition of cordial is "tending to revive, cheer, or invigorate; warmth and friendliness; possessing a warm, sincere, and friendly nature." Cordials were given these descriptions because they serve to invigorate your health enough that you feel like being nice to other people. Many of the recipes in the chapter on cordials contain lemon balm. Make a chamomile–lemon balm cordial to settle your temper and your tummy.

Lemon balm is a tea that children will drink; it keeps away snotty noses and calms an upset child. Drink hot lemon balm tea for colds or make your own tension-tamer tea with lemon balm and oatstraw. In Germany, lemon balm is a standard tea prescribed for sleeping disorders. Drink it, fill your bathtub with it, or chop the fresh herb and put it in cream dips and fruit salads.

Regular use of lemon balm is not advised with hypothyroidism.

**PROJECTS:** herbal water, herbal drinks, herbal smoothies, herbal honey, herbal vinegar, herbal cordial, herbal pesto, herbal bath and foot soak

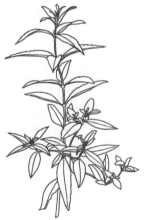

**COMMON NAME: lemon verbena**
**BOTANICAL NAME:** *Aloysia triphylla*
**PART USED: leaf**
**GARDENING TIPS:** Lemon verbena likes sun and sandy, well-drained soil. It can withstand some hard frost, but the soil has to be kept somewhat warm with heavy mulching. This is a deciduous herb that loses its leaves and turns into a spindly stick that

doesn't look like much of anything all winter long. I have had many students tell me that they thought they killed their lemon verbena and were surprised to see budding leaves in the spring.

**PROPERTIES:** anti-inflammatory, antispasmodic, astringent, carminative, nervine

**USES:** Having introduced this plant to well over a thousand people, I will tell you that the main response this plant elicits is a big smile and a loud "Ahh." The closest thing to describe the feeling that happens within a group of people standing around lemon verbena is that it creates a moment of mild euphoria that includes cooing, crooning, and sighing. This effect is not something I read about in a book. I just kept noticing how happy people become when they smell lemon verbena in the garden or in their tea. What is a moment of stress reduction worth? Well, it isn't very scientific, but it feels vitally important to have an herbal ally that just helps you to take a deep breath, relax, and feel good if even for a moment. I have lemon verbena growing by my front door. When I come home, I squeeze a bit of the leaf, take a whiff, and ah, here I am, calming down and feeling at home.

A superb beverage herb, lemon verbena makes pleasant summer iced tea, spritzers, coolers, smoothies, popsicles, herb water, and lemonade. One of the best things you can do for your health and your pocketbook is to develop a knack for throwing together tasty drinks. We rely too heavily on packaged beverages that contain sugar and caffeine and are costly. Energy drinks are a multimillion-dollar industry that is concerned about sales, not your health.

The addiction to coffee and sweet caffeinated drinks has exploded in recent years. Excess caffeine and sugar eventually cause people to feel fatigued and run-down. Over time, we need to drink more and more caffeine to maintain the energy level that one cup used to provide. Let's turn this around and popularize delicious drinks made with herbal nervines and healing tonics. Reach for a drink that reduces stress and enhances overall wellness by nourishing your body and nervous system. Sustain your energy with mineral-rich, rejuvenating tonics instead of with sugar and stimulants that eventually lead to depletion.

We use lemon verbena all summer long in drinks and smoothies. It's cooling, calming, and cheering. Put a few sprigs in your drinking water, make summer lemon verbena–blueberry vinegar for barbecue marinades, and liven up your smoothies with lemon verbena tea. Dried, powdered lemon verbena adds a bouquet of flavor when added to flour for making pies, cakes, scones, muffins, cookies/biscuits, pancakes, and raw desserts.

**PROJECTS:** herbal water, herbal drinks, herbal smoothies, herbal honey, herbal vinegar, herbal cordial, herbal bath and foot soak

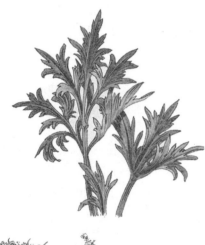

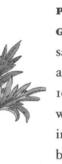

**COMMON NAME: mugwort**

**BOTANICAL NAME:** *Artemisia douglasiana*

**PART USED: leaf and flower**

**GARDENING TIPS:** Mugwort likes the sandy soil found at the edges of streams and riverbanks where it thrives to towering 10-foot (3-meter) stalks. It dies back in the winter and survives frost and snow to return in the spring. Mugwort withstands full sun but can also be found growing in semishade. It survives drought but will really flourish with at least moderate watering. This herb will attract ladybugs to your garden. In the fall, millions of ladybugs hang out in the mugwort patches where we live.

**PROPERTIES:** anthelmintic, antibacterial, antifungal, antispasmodic, bitter tonic, cholagogue, emmenagogue, nervine

**USES:** I had a massage therapy practice for twenty years, and the financial savings from making all of my own herbal massage oils was significant. I always had a half dozen oils available, and mugwort was one of the main oils requested by my clients. I would make up a big batch, put some of it in my kitchen, some of it next to the bathtub, and the rest of it stayed in the massage room. Mugwort is truly a massage therapist's ally; it warms and relaxes sore muscles so you don't have to work as hard! It increases blood circulation and has a deeply penetrating nature that helps relieve pain. Mugwort makes a luxurious oil that helps with lower back pain, menstrual cramps, and neck stiffness.

Mugwort has many personal and home care uses. Put dried mugwort into your grain and flour containers to repel moths and insects, add it to your food to inhibit parasites in your gut, and soak your feet in mugwort tea to get rid of athlete's foot. If you feel cold and congested, use some mugwort oil in your steamed vegetable dressing and then put a cup of the oil in your warm bath. Mugwort vinegar is delicious in salads and can also be applied with a washrag to the face for headaches. Mugwort vinegar relieves the itching from poison oak and is healing for bruises and sprains.

Mugwort opens up the sinuses, dispelling mucus and clearing the stagnation that can make colds and allergies such a miserable experience. It enhances mental clarity, clairvoyance, and self-awareness. It is a purifying and stimulating herb that activates intuition and memory. This aromatically pleasing herb is used as incense in ceremonies for healing. I burn it at the end of the day to clear out what I don't need and to help digest the day's experience.

The bitter flavor of mugwort makes it a digestive aid in assimilating nutrients. A sip of mugwort cordial before dinner not only enhances the nutrition of your food but also transforms the mundane into something special and ceremonial. Mugwort turns daily tasks into a meditation and communion with what you are doing. It is an illuminating herb that helps me to be more present and aware.

**PROJECTS:** herbal drinks, herbal smoothies, herbal honey, herbal vinegar, herbal cordial, herbal oil, herbal ghee, herbal bath and foot soak

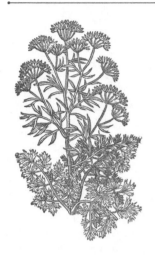

**COMMON NAME: mustard**

**BOTANICAL NAME: *Brassica hirta***

**PART USED: seed**

**GARDENING TIPS:** Our mustard grows in dry, disturbed soil and is not watered. It is one of the first flowers of spring, but once the heat sets in, it goes to seed and dries up. Mustard survives drought and poor soil in areas with mild to moderate winters. Eat some of the fresh spring greens and let the flowers go to seed. The recipes in this book refer to the yellow mustard seed.

**PROPERTIES:** analgesic, antibacterial, antioxidant, carminative, diuretic, expectorant, laxative, rubefacient

**USES:** Mustard is one of the herbs of my childhood. I have pictures of my mom and me sitting in golden fields of mustard flowers. Wading through the mustard fields was an annual ritual that was the signature of winter transforming into spring. Every March, the mustard unfolds throughout the hills in a brilliant carpet of yellow. The old-timers still go to the fields and harvest wild mustard greens for their spring meals. A timeless remedy, mustard seed is used to enhance digestion and disperses phlegm. Use extra mustard in your food if you have a wet cough; it will help to dissolve and expectorate excess mucus. Mustard seed is highly antioxidant, containing vitamins C and E, selenium, and omega-3 fatty acids. With our stressful lives and processed food consumption, we could use a little extra antioxidant support. Antioxidants slow the aging process, nurture a glowing complexion, and soften the effect of damaging free radicals. Foods rich in omega-3s help to reduce systemic inflammation that contributes to allergies, arthritis, and cancer. I eat a corn dog about once a year when we go to the local county fair. Do you think that drenching it in mustard might help the body process the damage from the trans fats in such foods?

When you use mustard seed, be careful not to boil it, as it becomes bitter. If you want the full flavor of mustard in cooking, soak it in room-temperature water for ten minutes before using. Soaking activates an enzyme that helps release the flavor, and heat destroys the flavor-producing enzymes. Mustard is also a good ingredient in salad dressings; along with stabilizing the emulsion process of fats and water, it adds a nice spike of flavor. A little mustard seed in your mayonnaise or salad dressing stabilizes the oil emulsion and prevents separation, giving you a nice, smooth product.

One of the strongest rubefacients in the herb world, mustard is a powerfully warming, penetrating, and moving herb. A strong circulatory stimulant, mustard brings blood to the surface of the skin, which enhances nutrient delivery to and waste removal from the body. If you are someone who runs around with chronically cold hands and feet, think about using a little mustard in your food, as it increases circulation throughout the body. Mustard used regularly can help reduce arthritic pain. For such a tiny seed, it is surprisingly vigorous in its ability to relieve pain, congestion, and stagnation.

**PROJECTS:** herbal honey, herbal vinegar, herbal cordial, herbal oil, herbal ghee, herbal pesto, herbal sprinkle, herbal bath and foot soak

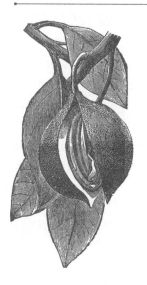

**COMMON NAME: nutmeg**

**BOTANICAL NAME:** *Myristica fragrans*

**PART USED: seed**

**GARDENING TIPS:** Nutmeg likes the hot, humid conditions of the tropics.

**PROPERTIES:** anthelmintic, antibacterial, anti-inflammatory, antispasmodic, carminative, expectorant, nervine, rubefacient

**USES:** Like many of the spices from the tropics, nutmeg is carminative and a superb digestive aid. It is traditionally used to treat diarrhea, nausea, vomiting, and digestive problems including gastroenteritis and malabsorption. Used in small amounts, it is the carminative of choice for seasoning winter foods. As the weather becomes colder, it is important to invite more herbal digestive aids into the diet. Digestive capacity dims with the light. When the sun goes down, so does your ability to absorb nutrients from your food. The level of vitality you experience as you navigate your day is directly proportional to how well you digest and absorb nutrients from your food. Try to eat your dinner earlier in the day as the seasons shift and darkness falls earlier in the evening. Eating late at night is a sure setup for indigestion and eventually more serious belly problems.

Nutmeg achieves higher status in daily household conversations during winter festivities. Consumption of nutmeg increases exponentially when the holiday season arrives, as sweets are produced en masse. It is the main spice in the illustrious beverage eggnog and is found simmering in mulled wines and ciders in living rooms across the country. Befriend nutmeg during the holidays; it mediates the effects of rich food, too many desserts, overeating, and late-night holiday feasting. Nutmeg is especially helpful with rich, dairy-filled foods. It is commonly added to cream and cheese sauces, egg dishes, and creamy desserts.

I keep powdered nutmeg in sprinkle formulas in my kitchen, but I don't let them sit around. Nutmeg is one of the spices that has a shorter shelf life once it is powdered. It contains oils that go rancid, so it is best to purchase whole nutmeg seeds and grate them fresh into food and drinks. If the seed turns dark brown or starts to get black spots, it has gone bad. I have fresh nutmeg on hand for grating into French toast and frittata egg batter. Nutmeg and star anise sprinkled on yams or baked winter squash is always a hit.

I have seen nutmeg help many people who suffer with insomnia. If you have trouble sleeping at night, stir ⅛ teaspoon (¼ g) of powdered nutmeg into very warm raw milk, and let it sit for a few minutes. Drink thirty minutes before going to bed to relax the muscles and nervous system. If you do well with dairy, this is a pleasant nightcap that promotes sound sleep. Nutmeg and cardamom added to warm almond milk make a rejuvenating drink for depletion and exhaustion. Nutmeg is toxic if taken in large doses, so nutmeg is added to food sparingly and in dashes.

**PROJECTS:** herbal water, herbal drinks, herbal smoothies, herbal honey, herbal vinegar, herbal cordial, herbal oil, herbal ghee, herbal sprinkle, herbal bath and foot soak

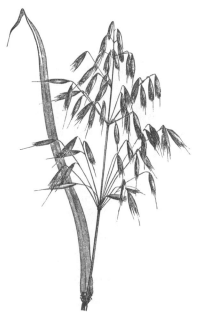

**COMMON NAME: oatstraw**

**BOTANICAL NAME:** *Avena sativa*

**PART USED: pod**

**GARDENING TIPS:** Oatstraw is an aggressive grain grass that grows in abundance everywhere I look. It tolerates full sun or shade. Oatstraw will grow with just the rainfall, but if you want a longer harvesting period, water it.

**PROPERTIES:** alterative, demulcent, nervine, nutritive, tonic, vulnerary

**USES:** I grew up playing in fields of oatstraw. Every open space and hill in sight was covered with it. When first beginning my herbal studies, I attended classes on the east coast. The herbalists in New York were talking about the indispensable uses of this marvelous grass called oatstraw that grew wild on the west coast. I was stunned to find out that the grass I rolled around in since the time I could walk held such high status in the herbal world. Oatstraw is all around one of the best herbs to help counteract the effects of a stressful lifestyle. It doesn't take the place of sleep, but it definitely helps with irritability, anxiety, nervousness, and exhaustion associated with stress.

Anxiety and stress have a debilitating effect on all parts of the body. Incorporating nervines into your food routine is one of the gifts of knowing how to use herbs to support your everyday lifestyle. Drinking tonic teas and using adaptogen and nervine herbs can just be what we come to expect, like lemonade in the summer and hot chocolate in the winter. Oatstraw is full of minerals and trace minerals and vitamins A and B. Its mild flavor puts it at the top of the list to use as a base tea for specialty drinks.

The stressors of life seem to come in waves, and some waves are bigger than others. Riding them out is both a challenge and an art. Plunging into the depths of the ocean is something that happens occasionally as part of the cycle of life, but be sure to surround yourself with loving people and drink your nervines so you don't stay down for too long. When life is transforming you in unexpected ways, use oatstraw to reinforce your vitality.

Oatstraw blends into an inviting tea with a mild and sweet taste that most everyone enjoys drinking. The results of working with this herb aren't noticeable overnight. Using oatstraw over time can help you to feel calmer, more grounded and centered, and definitely more capable of adjusting to your environment. I love the revitalizing feeling that comes with drinking oatstraw on a regular basis. It is gentle yet strong, soothing yet protective.

**PROJECTS:** herbal drinks, herbal smoothies, herbal vinegar, herbal cordial, herbal bath and foot soak

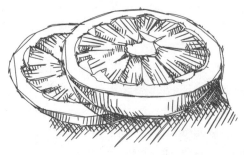

**COMMON NAME: orange peel**

**BOTANICAL NAME:** *Citrus sinensis*

**PART USED: peel**

**GARDENING TIPS:** Orange trees grow well in temperatures from 50 to 100°F (10 to 38°C). Sun and above-freezing temperatures are what you look for. Orange trees thrive in places like Texas and Florida.

**PROPERTIES:** Anti-inflammatory, antispasmodic, bitter tonic, cardiovascular tonic, carminative, expectorant, nervine

**USES:** Wait! Don't throw away those orange peels! Eat your orange, and then break the peel up into dime-size pieces. Fresh orange peels are delicious in herb waters. Add them to soups and stews or slow cook them with chicken or duck. Grate fresh orange peel into cookies/biscuits and breads or add a zesty flavor to sweets and desserts. After you have gotten your fill of fresh orange peels, let them sit out at room temperature on a screen until they are crispy. Once dried, store them in a jar in your spice cabinet. You now have a satisfying and revitalizing ingredient to use in your meal preparations throughout the year.

Orange peel not only adds a nice flavor to your food, but it also makes a very good-tasting tea. Orange, tangerine, and mandarin peel teas are traditionally used for coughs that are due to excessive phlegm in the lungs. It is a good tea to drink if you have lots of mucus, chronic chest congestion, or a wet cough. Citrus peels are considered a valuable medicinal herb and are a popular ingredient in many Chinese medicine tonics.

Citrus peels are loaded with vitamin C and pectin. Pectin, which is also abundant in apples, is a carbohydrate that feeds the beneficial bacterial in your gastrointestinal tract. Yes, your gut is full of creepy-crawly bacteria. You are a walking colony of bugs, an apartment complex for hundreds of different types of living organisms that can only be seen with a microscope. This beneficial microflora complements the immune system, helps us digest nutrients, and keeps pathogenic bacteria in check. Our daily wellness and vitality is intricately connected to the health of our gut bugs. Feed your bugs. When you eat sugar-ridden foods, you feed the bacteria that make you sick. When you eat orange peels, you feed the beneficial bacteria that keep you healthy. Don't throw away that orange peel!

A delicious addition to winter meals, orange peel chases away mucus and wards off colds and flu with its antibacterial, antifungal, and antiviral properties. Orange peels also help with sluggish digestion and are effective for treating gas, bloating, and nausea.

Most people throw away this part of their orange-eating experience because they just aren't aware of how beneficial the orange peels are. Its nature's giveaway; you get a free packet of delicious tea every time you eat an orange. Orange peels can be used in cooking in a surprising number of ways. Make an orange peel–rose hip sprinkle and put it in your smoothies and quinoa salad, or just have orange peels on hand to flavor other teas. Make an orange peel paste by powdering dried orange peels and adding just enough olive oil to make a paste to spread on fish before cooking.

**PROJECTS:** herbal water, herbal drinks, herbal smoothies, herbal honey, herbal vinegar, herbal cordial, herbal oil, herbal ghee, herbal sprinkle, herbal bath and foot soak

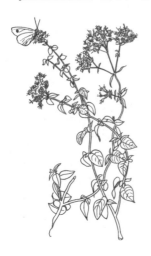

**COMMON NAME: oregano**

**BOTANICAL NAME: *Origanum vulgare***

**PART USED: leaf and flower**

**GARDENING TIPS:** Oregano does well with full sun and somewhat dry soil. It can winter over in hard frosts and then grows all spring, summer, and fall.

**PROPERTIES:** Antibacterial, antifungal, antioxidant, antispasmodic, antiviral, carminative, emmenagogue, expectorant, nervine

**USES:** Thousands of years ago, the Greeks gave this plant its name, "oregano," meaning mountain joy. Would you like more mountain joy in your life? There are plenty of reasons to put mountain joy into your food. Possessing strong antiviral, antibacterial, and antifungal properties, oregano keeps away everything that doesn't belong in our bodies. Oregano vinegar can be applied to athlete's foot; infused oregano oil can be applied to other fungus-infested areas of the body that we don't really need to specify here. Oregano is used in food preservation to deter food-borne pathogens. Sprinkled into your meals, oregano keeps unfavorable bacteria and parasites at bay. Adding oregano to your cuisine is good preventive health care.

An oregano foot soak helps to sweat out a cold. Oregano in your spaghetti sauce provides antioxidant nutrients and an oregano tea pacifies respiratory problems. Like thyme, oregano contains thymol, which is highly antiseptic and expectorant and helps to ease lung congestion. It is also rich in rosmarinic acid, which facilitates healing of bronchial inflammation. Oregano is traditionally used to treat spasmodic coughs, bronchitis, and excess phlegm. If you have a cough with thick secretions, you will benefit from a simple oregano tea.

If someone is catching a cold, before you run to the store, open your cupboard of kitchen cures. There have been numerous times that I have brewed teas from the spice cupboard to nip a cold in the bud. If you are visiting someone and notice that they are getting sick and not doing anything about it, enlighten them to the enormous possibilities sitting just inside their kitchen cabinet.

Oregano is high in vitamins A, C, and K, as well as iron, calcium, and manganese. Add minced fresh oregano to salads, tacos, and all foods that are garnished with lettuce. Culinary oregano oil adds a distinctive flavor that completes all tomato and bean dishes. Oregano and basil ghee is a sumptuous sautéing medium for red pasta sauces, and oregano oil will liven up any meat marinade. Do not mistake the infused herbal oils described in this book with the popular essential oil of oregano found in the stores.

**PROJECTS:** herbal smoothies, herbal honey, herbal vinegar, herbal cordial, herbal oil, herbal ghee, herbal pesto, herbal sprinkle, herbal bath and foot soak

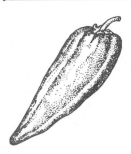

**COMMON NAME: paprika**

**BOTANICAL NAME:** *Capsicum annuum*

**PART USED: fruit**

**GARDENING TIPS:** Paprika adapts to different regions, but it thrives in warm weather. It does not like extended frost and grows in warm, dry climates in full sun. It likes well-tended garden beds with good water drainage and moist soil.

**PROPERTIES:** analgesic, antibacterial, anti-inflammatory, antioxidant, cardiovascular tonic, carminative, circulatory stimulant

**USES:** I love paprika; sweet paprika gives you the splendid flavor of a chile pepper without all the heat. Paprika ranges in flavor from mild and sweet to hot and pungent depending on processing methods and growing conditions. There are many varieties of paprika, so look for the cooler, sweet Hungarian paprika. If you want a hot pepper, then use cayenne. Paprika permeates your food with a full-bodied flavor that brings everyone back for seconds. We keep paprika on the table in a miniature bowl and sprinkle it onto practically all our dinner foods, and we use it much more frequently than salt. My son sprinkles it on rice, vegetables, and pizza!

Packed full of beneficial nutrients, paprika is high in vitamin C and contains the important antioxidant nutrient beta-carotene. Its flavonoid content has paprika weighing in as an important substance for the cardiovascular system. High-flavonoid spices are tonic to the heart, reducing the risk of heart disease by protecting the capillaries, veins, and the entire cardiovascular system. They help to prevent atherosclerosis by inhibiting the deposit of cholesterol on arterial walls. When there is a decrease in the integrity of collagen matrix of the arterial wall, it results in cholesterol being deposited there. If the matrix remains strong, the plaque won't stick. Paprika's red flavonoids increase the integrity of collagen structure in blood vessel walls, supporting cardiovascular health. I am betting on it as an antiaging serum. I will let you know how it works.

Adding flavonoid-rich foods to your diet also helps calm the inflammatory histamine response that plagues people with seasonal allergies. Spice up your life, give a lift to your health, and try adding paprika to your meals on a regular basis. I am simply addicted to this bright orange powder. Instead of reaching for the salt at mealtimes, try paprika instead.

Go beyond goulash and use paprika to enhance almost any salad or dinner meal. My mother's deviled eggs and macaroni salad was not complete unless doused with paprika before serving. The subtle yet rich and full-bodied flavor of paprika augments any fish, infuses well into oil, and can be drizzled onto breads, any egg dish, and tuna melts. One of the most consumed spices in the world, paprika captures your taste buds when added to soups and chowders. I put paprika on corn on the cob instead of salt and pepper. I have a lazy Susan full of herbal oils. The one I use most is a combination of paprika, coriander, cumin, and star anise. It turns anything into a gourmet creation.

**PROJECTS:** herbal honey, herbal vinegar, herbal cordial, herbal oil, herbal ghee, herbal pesto, herbal sprinkle

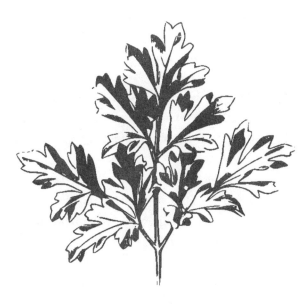

**COMMON NAME: parsley**
**BOTANICAL NAME:**
*Petroselinum crispum*
**PART USED: leaf**
**GARDENING TIPS:** Parsley likes full sun or partial shade and regular watering. When we have light frost years, I can eat from my parsley plant well into the winter. I have found that parsley does better after deep fertilizing with rich compost and worm castings. It prefers a rich, moist soil with good drainage.

**PROPERTIES:** anti-inflammatory, antioxidant, antispasmodic, aperient, diuretic, emmenagogue, nutritive, tonic

**USES:** My grandmother didn't teach me a lot about herbs, but she put parsley on our plate at dinner, and whenever we ate at a restaurant she made us eat the parsley. She said that it was the healthiest thing on the plate. Since most lunches at her house consisted of Velveeta cheese and white bread sandwiches, she was right.

I use both curly and flat-leaf parsley interchangeably. Flat-leaf has a little stronger flavor that I prefer, but they both can be used in the same way. You are sprinkling your food with vitamins and minerals when you put parsley in your lunch. Parsley is a nutrient-dense herb full of vitamins A and C, iron, calcium, and magnesium. It is rich in vitamins, chlorophyll, and flavonoids, making this mild-tasting herb an overall tonic for health and wellness. Chop it into grain, bean and pasta salads, or put into lettuce mixes and steamed greens. In the summer, parsley and dandelion leaf are the main herbs in my green drinks. When summer's harvest gives so much parsley that even I can't drink it all, I make Scarborough Fair vinegar with fresh parsley, sage, rosemary, and thyme. Its bounty of essential nutrients graces salads all summer long.

Parsley is anti-inflammatory. It inhibits the histamine reaction, making it a good herbal tea to drink when you have allergies or a runny nose. More than a garnish, parsley is an effective remedy for PMS symptoms including cramps, headaches, and water retention.

Parsley is high in chlorophyll, and it is a gentle diuretic helping to detoxify waste from the body. The American Center for Disease Control and Prevention has released recent studies showing that the average American now walks around with up to two hundred chemicals and twenty-one pesticides in their bloodstream that weren't there one hundred years ago. Eating herbs that can help the body rid itself of toxins turns out to be big medicine. Don't underestimate the health benefits of the simple parsley garnish.

**PROJECTS:** herbal water, herbal drinks, herbal smoothie, herbal vinegar, herbal oils, herbal ghee, herbal pesto, herbal sprinkle, herbal bath

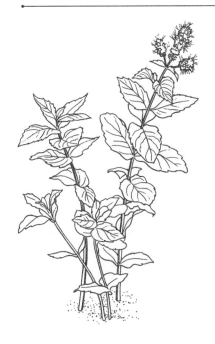

**COMMON NAME:** peppermint
**BOTANICAL NAME:** *Mentha piperita*
**PART USED:** **leaf and flower**
**GARDENING TIPS:** Full sun gives you the best-tasting peppermint. Keep it moist, but be careful where you plant it. Peppermint sends out invasive runners and can choke out the rest of your garden.
**PROPERTIES:** antibacterial, antifungal, antispasmodic, antiviral, carminative, cholagogue, nervine
**USES:** Peppermint is the best herb I have found to counteract the afternoon slump. It opens the sinuses and clears the head. Do you lose your memory after lunch? You have had your lunch, rested a bit, but you just can't seem to get your chi back up into your brain? Maybe it is time to take the rest of the day off, but if that is not an option, drink peppermint tea instead. Peppermint drinks help to increase mental clarity, and I drink them in the afternoon instead of coffee.

Peppermint is high in calcium, magnesium, potassium, and other beneficial nutrients. Making water-based drinks is one of the best ways to assimilate the nutrition that is available in peppermint. Start with just adding it to your drinking water, or make a strong peppermint tea and use it in smoothies and lemonade. Add sprigs of it to your pesto and green drinks and add powdered peppermint to meatballs and meat rubs for red meat. It is a nutrient-dense herb that you can have all kinds of fun with in the kitchen. Whatever you eat, peppermint will help you to digest it more efficiently, freeing up your body's energy to spend on doing whatever it is that you love to do.

When he was three years old, my son started picking peppermint and asking me to make a tea with it for him. Whenever he feels a little upset or has a tummyache, he asks for peppermint tea. Children love the smell of peppermint tea. For young children, the taste can be a little strong, so make a drink of half tea and half water. It eases stomach problems, calms the nerves, and fights off colds.

Most people associate peppermint with tea and candy. Peppermint candies served after dinner are a remnant of herbal knowledge from a time when people used peppermint to settle the digestive system after a heavy dinner. Peppermint is a wonderful garnish for summer foods. Mince fresh peppermint and make a confetti for fresh fruit, melon salad, or yogurt desserts. Peppermint goes well with rose petals and lemon balm for summer punch and spritzers. Spray peppermint vinegar on ants, and they will leave your kitchen.

Peppermint is not recommended for individuals with hiatal hernias or acute gallstones.

**PROJECTS:** herbal water, herbal drinks, herbal smoothie, herbal honey, herbal vinegar, herbal cordial, herbal oil, herbal ghee, herbal pesto, herbal sprinkle, herbal bath and foot soak

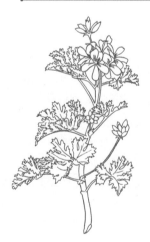

**COMMON NAME: rose geranium**

**BOTANICAL NAME:** *Pelargonium graveolens*

**PART USED: leaf and flower**

**GARDENING TIPS:** I love brushing up against this herb, releasing the aroma from the leaves as I walk around my house. I have it planted in all areas of our herb gardens. Its most uninhibited growth is in the area near the creek with the sandiest soil. It doesn't get as much water there, but it loves the rich, porous soil. Rose geranium likes moderate sun and also does well in full sun. Plant this herb in the walkway to your front door and next to where you park your car or your bike so that the scent surrounds you as you arrive home.

**PROPERTIES:** antibacterial, anti-inflammatory, astringent, hemostat, nervine, vulnerary

**USES:** If by some chance you don't feel like eating or drinking your rose geranium, the next best thing is to put it into your bathtub. Chop up the fresh herb and put an entire bundle in your bath while you draw the water. Basically you are making a big tub full of rose geranium tea in which to soak your body. Rose geranium is anti-inflammatory and mildly astringent, providing the perfect medium to tighten skin, reduce aggravated skin problems, and provide you with a radiant complexion. Externally, rose geranium treats bug bites, stings, sores, wounds, hemorrhoids, rashes, and bruises.

Rose geranium is known for being harmonizing, calming, relaxing, nourishing, replenishing, revitalizing, and uplifting. This plant makes me happy. I have it planted all around because for the few seconds that I smell it, I feel a sense of peace. Everything else leaves, and in that moment of being flooded with the essence of rose geranium, I feel content. A minute later my life rushes back in, but I figure if I take several rose geranium oasis breaks a day, it adds up.

I love fresh rose geranium tea, and it is a favorite honey spread in our house. Rose geranium is the perfect embellishment for fresh fruit salad, and it also makes a favorable sore throat gargle. It has a cooling and decongesting effect and finds its way into our lemonade, party drinks, and punches all summer long. It is also a nervine, dispensing a soothing and uplifting affect when stress and tension have taken over. Luxuriate in the refuge of your bathtub filled with rose geranium. Sip it, mince it into summer watermelon salad, drink rose geranium–orange peel punch, spread rose geranium–lavender butter on bread, and drizzle rose geranium honey on fruit desserts. It is truly the punctuation in summer's jubilee of fresh food.

I am not much of a cake and cookie baker, but I have friends who put several tablespoons of powdered rose geranium and lemon verbena into pound cake, shortcake, sponge cake, upside-down cake—any cake you can think of. We have a large celebration and herbal potluck at the end of my yearlong herbal studies course. One year, a student made lavender and rose geranium white cake with rose geranium–cream cheese frosting. It was decorated with lavender, rose geranium, rosemary, and calendula flowers. It was a showstopper, the ultimate herbal cake.

**PROJECTS:** herbal water, herbal drinks, herbal smoothies, herbal honey, herbal vinegar, herbal cordial, herbal pesto, herbal bath and foot soak

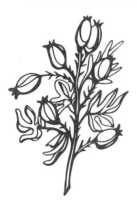

**COMMON NAME: rose hip**

**BOTANICAL NAME: *Rosa spp.***

**PART USED: hip**

**GARDENING TIPS:** If you want to harvest rose hips from your rosebush, don't cut the flowers from the bush. Simply let the flowers die on the plant, and they will turn into rose hips. Harvest the hips when they turn a deep orange or red and begin to get a little soft, which is usually after the first frost but before too much rain. Pick the hips. Halve them, scrape out the seeds and the hairs, and use the rose hip skins either fresh or dried in your herbal cooking.

**PROPERTIES:** antibacterial, anti-inflammatory, antioxidant, antispasmodic, aperient, astringent, carminative, nutritive, tonic

**USES:** We keep rose hip powder on the table right next to the salt. Its nutrient richness gives it claim to a central place at our table. Rose hips are recognized as one of the highest plant sources of vitamin C and have historically been used to treat scurvy. They are loaded with vitamins and minerals, and their carminative properties aid in the absorption of nutrients. Rose hips have a sweet, tart taste that adds a fizz of flavor to many varieties of foods. I like them sprinkled on rice and scrambled eggs. Rose hip honey is a staple food in our cupboard; we use it for baking, and it is delicious on pancakes. This is an herb that has superfood status and is easy to incorporate into daily meals.

Rose hips' anti-inflammatory flavonoids help to protect the gastrointestinal mucous membrane from the inflammation that is a rampant side effect of eating processed and pesticide-contaminated foods. Chemicals, preservatives, allergic reactions to denatured foods, and chlorinated water all have an irritating effect on the mucosal lining of the digestive tract. Excessive use of over-the-counter medications and antibiotics has also contributed to the epidemic of inflamed gut syndromes. People are becoming chronically ill at younger ages, and the soothing and restorative properties of rose hips are a relieving balm for the chronic digestive illnesses that burden our society.

Rose hips are a powerhouse of vitamins and minerals, making them an indispensable culinary medicine and tonic. If you don't currently use rose hips, just put some in a salt shaker and start shaking them into your breakfast. Many herbs side one way or the other with either savory or sweet foods, but rose hips run the gamut. Whether added to breakfast, lunch, or dinner, from raw foods to meat stew, rose hips have a welcoming taste and are full of healthful nutrients.

**PROJECTS:** herbal drinks, herbal smoothies, herbal honey, herbal vinegar, herbal cordial, herbal oils, herbal ghee, herbal sprinkle, herbal bath and foot soak

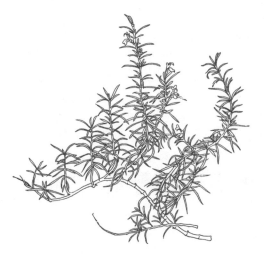

**COMMON NAME: rosemary**

**BOTANICAL NAME:** *Rosemarinus officinalis*

**PART USED: leaf and flower**

**GARDENING TIPS:** I have ten rosemary bushes that are about 3 feet (90 cm) wide by 4 feet (120 cm) tall in my garden. That is a lot of rosemary! Another Mediterranean native, it likes warm temperatures and lots of sun, but it also loves the moisture of a coastal environment. It does well in areas that have lots of sun and fog. Planting rosemary in your garden will bring the bees.

**PROPERTIES:** antibacterial, antifungal, antioxidant, antispasmodic, carminative, cholagogue, circulatory stimulant, emmenagogue, nervine, rubefacient

**USES:** I can never get enough of this plant. Rosemary improves circulation, relieves headaches, and is calming to the nervous system. The dark green leaves and the bright blue flowers of the rosemary ask us to stop and behold their beauty and healing power. I love drinking rosemary tea but most of all I enjoy putting several fresh sprigs of rosemary into my bath. Rosemary is an invigorating herb that gets everything in my body moving! If I feel a little sluggish, fatigued, or down-and-out, a rosemary bath shifts things to a new place. It is so uplifting that even just one bath with rosemary helps me to approach my life with a new perspective.

Drinking rosemary tea in the morning especially during the fall and winter really helps to stimulate circulation, bringing energy to the brain and all parts of the body. I think it is a good coffee substitute for people who use coffee to get their blood moving in the morning. Rosemary is much more subtle, but it has a good blood-moving effect. Rosemary is an invigorating herb that enhances memory and lifts the spirit. Traditionally this herb is used to reduce fatigue and enhance mental clarity. I hate to think of where I would be without this plant.

Studies show that rosemary is effective in slowing the growth of several bacteria that are involved in food spoilage. Rosemary has proven more effective in food preservation than many common food preservative additives. So if you are marinating or cooking up some meat, do what people have done for thousands of years with this herb: wrap the meat in rosemary.

Of course I add lots of fresh rosemary to my meals. I not only use it in marinades and sauces, but I also mince it finely and add it to salads and sprinkle it on rice, meat, and fish dishes. We have discovered that we like lots of rosemary with potatoes. We top baked potatoes with chives and minced rosemary, an excessive amount of rosemary goes into potato salads, and tons of rosemary and garlic are added to mashed potatoes.

I put a sprig of fresh rosemary in chardonnay about thirty minutes prior to drinking it at dinner. When rosemary is in bloom, garnish salads with the beautiful blue flowers and put them into the water that you drink during the day.

Did you know that rosemary is a great hair tonic? Just make three or four cups of rosemary tea before you take your next bath. Drink one cup and then pour the rest on your head! It stimulates circulation to your scalp, helps with dandruff, and makes your hair shiny. You can also make an extra cup of tea and gargle with it if you have any canker sores or inflammation in your gums. Now that is a multipurpose body care product.

**PROJECTS:** herbal water, herbal drinks, herbal smoothies, herbal honey, herbal vinegar, herbal cordial, herbal oil, herbal ghee, herbal pesto, herbal sprinkle, herbal bath and foot soak

---

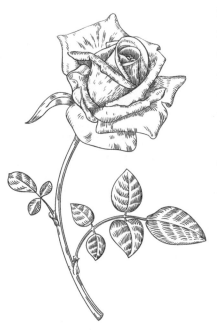

**COMMON NAME: rose petal**

**BOTANICAL NAME: *Rosa spp.***

**PART USED: flower petal**

**GARDENING TIPS:** Entire books, websites, organizations, societies, clubs, and magazines are dedicated to the art of growing roses. You need well-fertilized, well-draining soil with lots of sun. Roses also like access to circulating air. Don't grow them in a closed-in area. There are more than ten thousand varieties of cultivated roses. Choose rose stock that has already acclimated to the area where you live.

**PROPERTIES:** alterative, antibacterial, anti-inflammatory, aperient, astringent, nervine, nutritive, tonic

**USES:** People have surrounded themselves with roses but have forgotten that their blossoms are useful for more than bouquets. There are hundreds of ways to use rose petals, and extolling the healing virtues of roses is something that I love to do. I teach a class called Roses Forever where we spend an entire day talking about the remarkable characteristics of roses. Florist roses are routinely cultivated with pesticides, so look for organically grown roses.

Roses are a valuable medicine, food, and cosmetic ingredient and of course have a traditional reputation of being associated with love and beauty. Start by eating them! Chop up your fresh rose petals and put them on your sandwiches and salads. First I smell a rose, and then I take a bite out of it! My five-year-old son follows in his mom's footsteps. We walk around the block sniffing and nipping at the roses in our neighborhood. He takes a whiff, and then he takes a bite!

Rose petals are cooling and can be put in teas and drinks to temper summer's swelter. They are also an effective topical anti-inflammatory; gargle with rose petal tea for a sore throat, take a rose petal bath to help with hemorrhoids, and apply rose petal honey to acne or irritated facial skin.

Roses really are an all-around beauty treatment herb with an exceptional affinity for healing the skin. Their sweet and cooling nature gives them an excellent reputation as a topical remedy for heat-related conditions and heat exposure. Take a rose petal bath to console red and rashy skin. Rose petal vinegar is astringent to ulcerative skin conditions and helps with troublesome inflammation including acne, thread veins, varicose veins, capillary damage, scars, burns, and wrinkles. Apply rose petal vinegar to cool down sunburns or calm heat-induced headaches.

Roses tighten and heal skin tissue and are beneficial for all skin types. Rose remedies prevent infection of minor skin abrasions and cuts and reduce the swelling associated with bruises and sprains. Cleansing and toning, rose petals prevent and smooth out wrinkles, clear blemishes, and heal boils and sores. They shrink capillary redness and inflammation and have a cooling and soothing effect throughout the body. Use rose petals in facial masks, steams, body wraps, therapeutic baths and foot soaks.

As an effective nerve tonic, roses exert an uplifting and restorative influence on the nervous system. Nerve tonics enhance our mental function, moderate reactivity to our environment, and improve our ability to sleep. Roses have a calming effect and help with anxiety, restlessness, and nervousness.

**PROJECTS:** herbal water, herbal drinks, herbal smoothies, herbal honey, herbal vinegar, herbal cordial, herbal ghee, herbal pesto, herbal sprinkle, herbal bath and foot soak

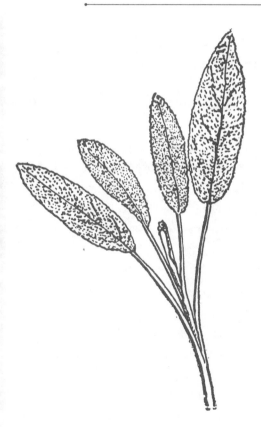

**COMMON NAME: sage**

**BOTANICAL NAME: *Salvia officinalis***

**PART USED: leaf**

**GARDENING TIPS:** Sage likes full sun, moderate water, and well-drained soil.

**PROPERTIES:** Antibacterial, anticatarrhal, antifungal, anti-inflammatory, antioxidant, antispasmodic, antiviral, astringent, carminative, nervine

**USES:** Once I was giving a talk about the medicinal qualities of sage, and a woman raised her hand and asked, "Do you mean Thanksgiving turkey stuffing sage?" Yes, turkey stuffing sage is what I am talking about. Take it out of the cupboard; you will now imbue your meals with it more than once a year. People use sage to accompany heavy meat feasts because it is an antidote to many of the problems that are associated with eating too much meat. The carminative properties help us to digest the meat, the antibacterial properties help to deter bacterial pathogens that may be growing in the meat, and its decongestant properties help to dispel congestion that many people develop from eating large portions of meat.

Sage is the ultimate kitchen medicine. Everyone has it in their spice cabinet, and its healing applications are notable enough to give this herb the family name "Salvia," which means "healthy and whole" in Latin. Sage is a much more versatile herb than we usually give it credit for. If the medicine chest is lacking, open up the spice drawer and make a cup of sage tea. It is brimming with minerals and holds a place in the forefront of all cold and flu remedies. Sage tea helps rid the body of coughs. Add more sage to your food if people around you are coughing and sneezing. Gargle with sage vinegar for laryngitis, a sore throat, or receding gums, and add sage to your sauces and marinades as part of your winter cold-prevention program. I put one sage leaf in my summer morning smoothie and add sage to my evening bath to keep sickness away.

Don't overlook the nervine qualities of sage. Life's pace just seems to be moving faster and faster, with more images to process, more information to assimilate, and too many technological devices with which to send and pick up messages. Nervine herbs bolster the nervous system so that relaxation is more within reach. While fending off colds, sage tea can also help bring on a pleasant night's sleep.

I love sage blossoms. The beautiful purple blooms make a nice cut flower. I harvest several bunches and put them in a vase in the center of the dining room table. What I noticed with using sage this way is that it energetically clears the space. It is almost like an acupuncture treatment for the room. Its antibacterial, aromatic oils kill airborne bacteria, and the fresh smell brings a sense of clarity.

**PROJECTS:** herbal drinks, herbal smoothies, herbal honey, herbal vinegar, herbal cordial, herbal oil, herbal ghee, herbal pesto, herbal sprinkle, herbal bath and foot soak

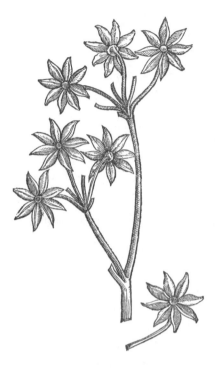

**COMMON NAME: star anise**

**BOTANICAL NAME: *Illicium verum***

**PART USED: pod and seed**

**GARDENING TIPS:** Star anise is cultivated in tropical and subtropical environments in shady to partially shady areas. Star anise is grown mainly in China and Vietnam.

**PROPERTIES:** antibacterial, anticatarrh, antispasmodic, antiviral, aperient, carminative, diuretic, expectorant, galactagogue

**USES:** This star-shaped seedpod is a warm and pungent herb with a powerful flavor. A single star is enough to flavor one soup or stew. Alive with hints of clove and licorice, this warming spice dispels abdominal cramping, burping, bloating, constipation, gas, indigestion, and stomachaches.

If you experience gas and bloating after meals, combine equal parts powdered ginger, black pepper, and star anise; make a sprinkle or a honey with the mixture; and use it in your cooking. The star anise activates digestive enzymes, helping you to assimilate heavy foods, especially fats and meats. Small amounts of star anise in condiments and sprinkles tucked into your meals will accelerate the sluggish digestion that is a root cause of innumerable ailments.

We have an epidemic of digestive problems, and the top-selling drugs are for indigestion complaints. Our overuse of antibiotics since the 1940s has resulted in digestive problems that have become generational. With this in mind, don't underestimate the value of adding carminatives to your food; they enhance the absorption of nutrients, supporting your body in building healthier cells and organs. When your cells are healthier, you experience more energy and creativity in your daily life. When our vitality is available to us for more than digesting food, we have more time to rejoice in all that life has to offer.

Shikimic acid is extracted from star anise and used in the production of the antiviral drug Tamiflu. Take advantage of the antiviral properties of star anise and keep a jar of these perfect multipointed seedpods next to your slow cooker. Put one or two pods into any slow cooker goulash. Not only will star anise hinder the flu, but it also helps to keep your lungs clear of the annoying mucus that can leave you susceptible to catching the flu. Star anise is both anti-catarrhal and expectorant; these features work together to liquefy thick mucus so it can be more easily expelled.

**PROJECTS:** herbal water, herbal drinks, herbal smoothies, herbal honey, herbal vinegar, herbal cordial, herbal oil, herbal ghee, herbal sprinkle, herbal bath and foot soak

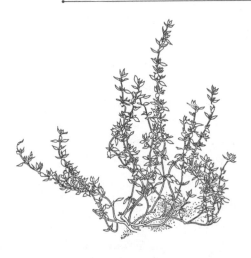

**COMMON NAME: thyme**

**BOTANICAL NAME: _Thymus vulgaris_**

**PART USED: leaf and flower**

**GARDENING TIPS:** Thyme likes full sun, mulched warm soil, and moderate watering. With a little attention to amending the soil with rich compost, you can grow enough thyme to meet all of your cooking needs.

**PROPERTIES:** anthelmintic, antibacterial, anticatarrh, antifungal, antiviral, antioxidant, antispasmodic, carminative, emmenagogue, expectorant, nervine

**USES:** Thyme improves all problems associated with the lungs and throat. It is one of our best respiratory remedies, as it expedites the healing of chronic and acute bronchial infection, spasmodic, wet coughs, chest colds, sore throats, hay fever, and sinus problems. The warming and drying nature of thyme comes to our rescue for moist, mucus-laden burdens that settle in the sinus and lungs. Thyme liquefies and clears congestion. Use it when you have lots of snot and a rattling cough. Swish a thyme tea gargle for sore throats and gum inflammation, take thyme honey to expel mucus, and cook with thyme oil to support respiratory health in general.

Thyme is full of minerals and trace minerals including iron. I always make note of herbs rich in iron, since women often need iron tonic support at various times in their lives. Drinking an iron-rich tea is beneficial after menstruation, during menopausal changes, and after childbirth. Take advantage of the easy-to-assimilate iron that is found in many kitchen herbs such as parsley, fenugreek, dandelion, peppermint, and thyme.

Thyme is a great culinary herb that can be added to many savory foods. It not only enhances the flavor of your supper, but eating it is also smart preventive medicine. It is a very strong antibacterial and antioxidant plant that keeps pathogenic bacteria from growing in your food. It helps to preserve meats and keeps oils from going rancid. Whip thyme and oregano into room-temperature butter just before putting it on Jerusalem artichokes or potatoes. It is delicious and also helps you to digest the starch in the root vegetables and the fat in the butter.

A mixture of powdered thyme, chives, parsley, rosemary, and celery seed sits on my kitchen table and is added to food as a salt substitute (see Garden Salt Substitute, page 243). Thyme is a wonderful carminative herb, stimulating the movement of energy, blood, and oxygen to the digestive tract. Add thyme to your food or add thyme honey to your after-dinner tea and take note of how well you digest what you have eaten. Thyme will dispel any gas, bloating, or indigestion that your food might cause. Ultimately we want to eliminate foods that cause gas, bloating, and digestive upset from our diets, but while you are figuring that one out, use more thyme.

You won't be the first person inspired to mix and match the savory delight of thyme with other herbs in accenting your gustatory adventures. Thyme is a principal ingredient in the centuries-old Benedictine liqueur. Follow in the footsteps of the Benedictine monks and formulate your own thyme cordial. Make Middle Eastern za'atar; a commonly used condiment comprised of thyme, sesame seeds, sumac, and salt. Create a personalized version of herbes de Provence, which traditionally includes thyme, fennel, rosemary, and bay leaf.

Across the globe, thyme has made its mark as a potent and indispensable ingredient. In the Caribbean, it is a vital addition to the well-known Jamaican jerk spice, which consists of brown sugar, thyme, allspice, garlic, cinnamon, and nutmeg. Travel to Egypt, and you won't be able to avoid spicing your foods with the ubiquitous dukka, a mixture of toasted sesame seeds, thyme, coriander, cumin, and black pepper. Thyme also permeates the spice mixtures used in the world-renowned cooking of New Orleans.

I would be remiss not to mention how much success I have witnessed with people using thyme foot soaks to pacify itchy fungal infections that often settle in the feet. Take advantage of thyme's broad spectrum of antibacterial and antifungal characteristics. Indulge yourself in its potent disinfectant action: stick your feet in it, or pour it into your winter soups. Just don't soak your feet in it and then put it into your soup!

**PROJECTS:** herbal water, herbal drinks, herbal smoothies, herbal honey, herbal vinegar, herbal cordial, herbal oil, herbal ghee, herbal pesto, herbal sprinkle, herbal bath and foot soak

---

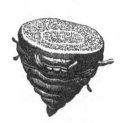

**COMMON NAME: turmeric**

**BOTANICAL NAME: *Curcuma longa***

**PART USED: root**

**GARDENING TIPS:** Turmeric is grown in tropical conditions and widely cultivated in India. You can purchase turmeric fresh at some Asian markets or buy it dried.

**PROPERTIES:** adaptogen, alterative, antibacterial, anti-inflammatory, antioxidant, carminative, cholagogue, hemostat, vulnerary

USES: This is another herb that holds an honorable place at the dinner table. When sprinkled onto food, its mild flavor enhances just about any savory dish. Since it is on the table, I have put it into foods that I would never have originally thought of adding it to. I love it in tuna salad, chicken salad, rice, pesto, eggs, bean salads, millet dishes, and sautéed vegetables. People who aren't on the herbal highway of life don't always like their food illuminated with a yellow glow, so just be a little more conservative when serving it to your friends and family members who are just getting into herbs. If you don't want to eat turmeric in your fish salad wrap, then make a turmeric paste with water and oil and apply it to your skin for fifteen minutes. It will leave your skin a little yellow for a short time, but the lasting radiance is worth it. Turmeric is a rejuvenating remedy for the skin and its restorative traits are reflected on spa menus and wellness resorts everywhere.

Turmeric has many specialties, including the ability to enhance immunity. It is full of antioxidants such as vitamins C and E, which are key nutrients in supporting the immune system. Turmeric slows the development of some cancer cells and stimulates immune cells that fight cancer. In addition to bolstering the immune system, clinical results attest to its antitumor and anticancer effects. Using this proven anticancer spice in your food is a valuable component in any basic health care plan.

The cholagogue properties of this sunshine-yellow root help increase the flow of bile, fortifying liver health. Turmeric is a recuperative tonic to liver cells, recharging their ability to process the excess toxins we are exposed to in our food and environment. Invigorating the production and flow of bile favorably influences the digestion of fats. Drizzle turmeric oil on your dinner to help you digest protein and fat and to absorb your minerals more efficiently.

If you are one of the growing numbers of people suffering from arthritic complaints, this is the spice to incorporate into your diet. Turmeric claims a long history of being taken to reduce rheumatic pain. It cools your joints and has been clinically proven to reduce the inflammation that contributes to arthritis. Inform yourself about the possible side effects of arthritis drugs, and that will be incentive enough to partner with turmeric. Try taking a teaspoon of turmeric-ginger honey twice a day to reduce joint inflammation.

Turmeric is not recommended for individuals with bile duct obstruction.

**PROJECTS:** herbal honey, herbal vinegar, herbal oil, herbal ghee, herbal pesto, herbal sprinkle, herbal bath and foot soak

---

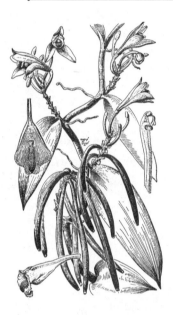

**COMMON NAME:** vanilla

**BOTANICAL NAME:** *Vanilla planifolia*

**PART USED: pod and seed**

**GARDENING TIPS:** Most of the world's supply of vanilla is grown in Indonesia and Mexico. Vanilla is a tropical orchid; it likes a warm, humid climate with lots of rain. Growing vanilla beans/pods is an extremely labor-intensive process. Each flower has to be individually pollinated, and curing the bean takes months of hand processing. No wonder this black, oily pod is one of the most expensive spices available. When purchasing vanilla, look for beans/pods that are supple, oily, and dark brown to black. Pass up any beans that are hard, dry, or light in color.

**PROPERTIES:** antioxidant, carminative, nervine

**USES:** The eclectic herbalists who practiced herbal medicine in the United States in the early twentieth century noted that vanilla was used for treating hysteria. The aroma of vanilla does have a calming and mildly euphoric effect on people. Its mood-enhancing fragrance has a soothing and pleasing charm whether it adorns ice cream or coffee drinks. It isn't just the ice cream but the vanilla in the ice cream that makes it such a delectable treat.

Very few studies have been conducted on the efficacy of vanilla uses for health issues. My friend from Mexico tells of her mother's uses of vanilla to help sharpen the mind and strengthen memory. I trust the empirical evidence of results noticed over time by mothers and grandmothers, even if it hasn't yet been proven by science.

The studies that have been conducted with vanilla center around its constituent, vanillin, which tests show has an inhibiting affect on the enzymatic activity of cancer cells. Extensive care is taken to potentiate the vanillin concentration in the pod to give vanilla its complex sweet aroma. Vanillin is proven to be highly antioxidant; all the more reason to use it in your culinary pursuits. Free radical damage from bad food, pollution, injury, and stress weaken the immune system and cause more rapid aging. Antioxidant spices have an antiaging effect. They neutralize free radicals and slow the aging process. Vanilla also has a calming influence, soothing physical and emotional tension that is fed by the pervasive undercurrent of stress that runs through so much of our lives. Nothing is more aging than excess stress, so make some vanilla honey and put it on your toast or add it to your tea.

Use the recipes in chapter 8 (Vanilla Cordial and Vanilla Spice Cordial, page 203) to make your own vanilla extract/essence. Avoid using imitation vanilla in your cooking; you don't need more chemicals in your life. Save some money and make your own high-quality vanilla extract, and you will use it more often. Customize your vanilla extract and add other herbs that complement vanilla, like cinnamon, nutmeg, clove, allspice, and orange peel. I have some vanilla cordial that is ten years old, and it just seems to get better as it ages. Try my luscious Love Potion Cordial (page 201), which reigns supreme for ceremonial toasts.

**PROJECTS:** herbal drinks, herbal smoothies, herbal honey, herbal vinegar, herbal cordial

PART THREE

# Herbal Recipes

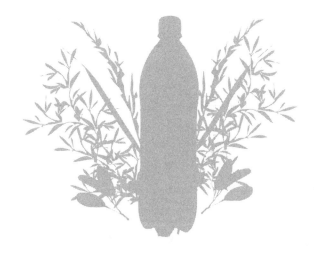

CHAPTER 3

# Herbal Waters

Herb waters are really nothing fancy, yet when you are served water garnished with herbs, you feel like special attention has been given to quench your thirst. I got in the habit of serving herb waters in the summer because it was just too hot to boil water for tea. If someone drops by and I don't have an herbal drink made for the day, I can quickly pick a few sprigs of herbs, chop a few slices of whatever fruit is in season, and put them into a pitcher of water. Guests are then offered a refreshment that is not only visually pleasing but also more satisfying than plain water.

The combinations of ingredients that can be added to water to make simple yet elegant drinks are endless. With fresh-picked herbs and fruit, the waters take on the flavor of each season, depending on what is ripe. People always comment about how they enjoy the herbs in the water. Sometimes I add a few dried spices, like a stick of cinnamon or a few allspice pods. We often think of presentation of the food on our plates. Herbed waters are my way of decorating drinks.

# GETTING STARTED

**SUPPLIES**

8-cup (2-L) pitcher

I like to collect pitchers for serving summer iced tea and herbed waters. I have antique glass pitchers, ceramic pitchers, and plastic picnic pitchers. The pitcher itself adds flair to the hospitality that I enjoy.

**INGREDIENTS**

filtered water

5 sprigs of fresh herbs

½ cup (93 g) thinly sliced fruit

dried spices

# MAKING AN HERBAL WATER

**METHOD**

1. Fill a pitcher with water.
2. Rinse freshly cut sprigs of herbs and add them to the water.
3. Thinly slice seasonal fruit and add the slices to the water.
4. Add a few dried spices, if desired.

**STORAGE**

Herb waters store in the refrigerator for several days. If you add fruit, the shelf life is shorter.

# RECICES

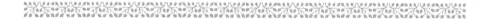

The combinations here are a result of years of our garden and fruit tree harvests. Rinse the sprigs of herbs before putting them into the water. Herbed water is subtle; you don't need a lot of ingredients. Just a few sprigs of herbs and a few slices or small scoops of fruit will do. Here are some combinations that my garden has presented.

basil and peppermint

basil and pomegranate

calendula and melon

calendula and rose petal

chamomile and kiwi

chamomile and plum

cinnamon and apricot

cucumber and peppermint

elder flower and lime

fennel seed and orange peel

lavender and plum

lavender, rose geranium, and lime peel

lavender and strawberry

lemon balm and cantaloupe/
  rockmelon

lemon balm and peach

lemon geranium and kiwi

lemon verbena and blueberry

orange peel and mint

peaches and clove

peppermint and apricot

peppermint and kiwi

peppermint and lemon

peppermint and orange

pine needle and lemon

rose geranium and rose petal

rose geranium and watermelon

rose petal and peppermint

rose petal and pomegranate

rose petal and strawberry

rosemary and peach

rosemary and persimmon

CHAPTER 4

# Herbal Drinks

Herbal drinks are healthful, delicious, and easy to make. I am evangelical when it comes to teaching children and adults how to make their own teas, drinks, sodas, and tea juices. Widespread consumption of high-sugar drinks has played a role in the startling increase in obesity and diabetes, which are among the top public health concerns in the United States. Obesity in children has increased almost 50 percent in the past forty years, and diabetes is currently escalating at an unprecedented rate in the United States. There are of course many other factors that contribute to these health risks, but let's put the conversation about sugar drinks and soda up front where it needs to be.

Our amazing human body constantly regenerates itself. New cells are made not just from what we eat but also from what we drink. Every time you take a drink, you have the opportunity to overwhelm your body with sugar and chemicals or to support and nourish it with minerals and nutrients. It all comes down to how good you want to feel each day and how healthy you want to be.

One important step toward optimum health is to just say no to soda. To begin with, the average soda contains more than 7 teaspoons (35 g) of sugar. Add artificial colors and sweeteners to the mix, and the question becomes, "Just what is it that I am feeding my body?"

Teenagers consume the most soda, but parents give sodas to small children and even infants. The pancreas in a small child's body has not matured enough to handle the sugar that floods the body when fed soda or pure fruit juice. If you give your children soda, you are increasing their risk of having health problems and gambling with diabetes. Please think twice before you offer soda to a child.

THE HERBAL KITCHEN

Soda is such a poor choice that I am continually surprised when it is the main beverage option on the child's menu and in the school vending machines. Soda contributes to diabetes, obesity, and tooth decay, and caffeinated sodas deplete calcium from the body. Not only are people still drinking sodas, but soda consumption has increased more than 40 percent in the last twenty years. We know it is bad for us, but we continue to drink it. As many of us lead busy lifestyles, we stray further and further away from the kitchen and forget how easy it is to devise creative, delicious homemade beverages.

I was raised with very little food, herb, or body literacy. By the fourth grade, I had become interested in what was labeled as "natural food." I knew I was on to something when my teacher demonstrated what cola could do. A fellow student brought his front tooth to school for show-and-tell. The teacher tied the tooth on a string and suspended it in a can of cola. Within two days, the tooth disintegrated. That classroom experiment had a major impact on me. I loved my family; why were they always drinking something that could dissolve teeth? Much to their dismay, after that day in class, I never stopped hassling them about drinking sodas. Get the sodas out of the schools, off the playgrounds, out of the lunch box, and off the child's menu. Just because we have a party doesn't mean we need to serve sodas. They don't really taste that great anyway; let go of the addiction. And don't be fooled by designer sodas. Look at the sugar content and avoid drinking anything with corn syrup or high-fructose corn syrup in it.

The good news is that healthful drinks are simple and really don't take much effort to make. In the time you wait in line at the store to buy the packaged drinks, you could have put together a week's worth of drinks at home. Take some time to think about and plan what you are going to drink instead of grabbing a soda. An added benefit to concocting your own beverages is that you can count on significant financial savings.

I hope you enjoy these healing drinks that are refreshing, full of ready-to-absorb nutrients, and easy to make. Let these recipes inspire you to drink your way to good health.

# GETTING STARTED

saucepan

glass jar with lid

strainer

8-cup (2-L) pitcher, preferably one with lid

## INGREDIENTS

### Herbs

Use fresh or dried herbs for making herbal drinks. We serve winter drinks warm and summer drinks at room temperature or slightly chilled. My favorite herbs to make our summer drinks with are burdock, chamomile, elder flower, lavender, lemon balm, lemon verbena, rose geranium, oatstraw, peppermint, and rose petals. We make winter teas with more warming herbs like astragalus, cinnamon, clove, elderberries, ginger, and rosemary. Make a tea with one herb or mix several together. Brew up your own favorite drinks and have a pitcher full in the summer or a pot warming on the stove in the winter.

### Fresh Fruit

Fresh, seasonal fruit is always preferred. The farmers' market is usually the place to find the best deals and the freshest harvest.

### Fruit Juice

Use whole fruit juice, not fruit juice with added sugar or high-fructose corn syrup. Read your labels. I cannot count how many times one of my clients has said, "Oh, I am drinking healthful cranberry juice," and then we read the label and the second ingredient listed is high-fructose corn syrup.

Be aware that fruit juice is also a high-sugar drink, even the 100 percent organic juices that advertise a profusion of health benefits. The fiber in fruit slows down the rate at which the sugar in the fruit is digested. When you drink straight fruit juice, the sugar in the fruit isn't buffered with the fiber, and the pancreas has to go into quick-response mode to release enough insulin to handle the undiluted sugar. Don't make the mistake of just trading soda for fruit juice. Whenever we drink fruit juice at our house, we cut it with at least one-half water. Especially avoid feeding 100 percent fruit juice to children on a regular basis. If you give your kids half juice and half water, they won't even know the difference.

If you are used to drinking sweet-tasting beverages, begin by adding just enough fruit juice to your tea so that it tastes good to you. Once you get comfortable with half juice and half tea, then you can continue to reduce the fruit juice. Our summer drinks are often a mixture of one-third herbal tea, one-third carbonated water, and one-third fruit juice. Sometimes we use less juice or none at all. After a while you find that you really don't even need that much fruit juice. The party drinks usually contain more fruit juice or carbonated water than everyday drinks. Summer drinks have more fruit ingredients than the winter drinks. Even when you add just a splash of juice, it is enough to give your drinks a refreshing and satisfying taste.

## Rose Water

Rose water is distilled from rose petals and adds an aromatic bouquet to your specialty drinks. Adding ½ cup (125 ml) of rose water to 4 cups (1 L) of tea is a good proportion to begin with. Rose water usually goes into punch-type teas for special occasions.

## Sweeteners

The nice thing about designing your own drinks is that you can control the sweetness, and over time, you can train your palate to crave less and less sugar. There are many things that you can use to sweeten your tea drinks. In addition to fruit and fruit juice, honey, herbal honey (see chapter 6), dehydrated cane juice, maple syrup, and stevia extract are the sweeteners of choice. Adding a splash of herbed or fruited vinegar is always nice. Recipes for herbal vinegars can be found in chapter 7.

## Carbonated Water

Carbonated water is an optional ingredient that satisfies soda drinkers. We use it to add a nice fizz to summer drinks.

# MAKING HERBAL DRINKS

The main ingredient in herbal drinks is herbal tea. You can drink the tea plain, or add a medley of other ingredients such as fresh fruit, fresh juice, carbonated water, or herbal honey.

To make delicious summer drinks, begin with a base recipe of equal parts herbal tea, organic fruit juice, and water or carbonated water. An easy way to start is to make 1 cup (250 ml) of tea and add 1 cup (250 ml) of juice and 1 cup (250 ml) of carbonated water. Chill and garnish with lemon or lime. After that becomes second nature, let yourself experiment with proportions, ingredients, and garnishes. Summer teas can be served plain, or you can mix in some honey or herbed honey. That might be enough to satisfy everyone. Add fruit juice if you are accustomed to sweeter drinks. If you enjoy carbonated drinks, add carbonated water just before serving. You will be amazed with the delicious cocktails you invent. The combinations within these guidelines are endless. You may be surprised at how much you enjoy your homemade concoctions.

## PROPORTIONS

1 tablespoon (15 g) dried ingredients per 1 cup (250 ml) of water
2 tablespoons (30 g) fresh ingredients per 1 cup (250 ml) of water

Dried herbs and spices are usually stronger than fresh ones. Fresh herbs contain water and take up more space. In general, I use up to twice the amount of fresh ingredients as dried. However, this is a general guideline, and each herb possesses different qualities that unveil themselves to you over time. If the recipe calls for multiple dried herbs, the total mixture of herbs is 1 tablespoon (15 g) of herbs added to each 1 cup (250 ml) of water. If the recipe calls for 1 cup (250 ml) of water and three herbs in the tea, put in 1 teaspoon (5 g) of each herb, which equals 1 tablespoon (15 g) in total. Avoid the mistake of putting 1 tablespoon (15 g) of each herb in the tea.

### METHOD #1: USING A TEA HOLDER OR BAG

1. Put 2 tablespoons (30 g) of dried herbs or 4 tablespoons (60 g) of fresh herbs into a mesh tea holder and put it into a teapot.

2. Pour 2 cups (500 ml) of boiling water over the top of the herbs and let steep for two hours.

3. Remove the tea holder. Enjoy your tea as is, reheated if desired, or add optional ingredients and serve hot or cold.

### METHOD #2: LOOSE HERBS

1. Place loose fresh or dried herbs and water into a covered saucepan. I use stainless steel Revere pots; glass and enamel pots also work well.

2. Over medium-high heat, bring water and herbs to a boil, and then immediately remove from the heat. Let herbs steep for one to two hours.

3. Using a metal strainer, remove the herbs from the tea and pour the tea into a teacup or pitcher. If you plan to drink the tea within a day, you can leave the herbs in the water if desired.

### METHOD #3: SUN TEA

1. Place herbs and water into an 8-cup (2-L) Mason jar.

2. Set it outside in the sun for a few hours. If it is a hot day, the herbs can also be steeped in room-temperature water on the counter for a few hours.

3. Strain tea (or not) and enjoy.

### STORAGE

Your herbal drinks usually have a shelf life of a couple of days. Herbal teas last for up to three days in the refrigerator. Put a lid on the tea container, as the tea can absorb odors and bacteria from the refrigerator. If the tea is left on the counter, it is usually good for one day, sometimes two, depending on the time of year and which herbs are in the tea.

If you use fresh fruit, depending on the type of fruit, it can start to ferment earlier. If you don't drink your brew right away, you can freeze it into Popsicle holders for ice pops or pour it into ice cube trays to make herbal ice cubes for adding to smoothies and drinks.

# RECITES

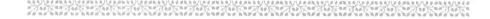

**COOL DRINKS**

Don't even walk down the soda aisle in the grocery store, skip ordering drinks at the restaurant, and enjoy your rousing homemade beverages. Here are some of my favorite summer drinks. They are time-tested crowd pleasers.

## APPLE-PEPPERMINT PLEASURE

*This is a summer staple at our house. The sweetness of the apples quench your thirst, and the peppermint cools the body. It is the perfect summer afternoon drink.*

2 cups (500 ml) peppermint tea

Fresh juice from 4 apples

Dash of powdered cinnamon

## ELDER FLOWER DELIGHT

*This recipe was developed one evening when a neighbor dropped by with a bag of freshly picked limes. I had a large pot of elder flower tea on the stove that my son had been drinking for his allergies. I added the fresh limes and other ingredients and turned our hay fever tea into a sumptuous dinner cocktail!*

2 cups (500 ml) elder flower–rose petal tea

¼ cup (60 ml) rose water

3 tablespoons (65 ml) maple syrup

¼ (60 ml) cup fresh lime juice

## GINGER-BERRY JUICE

*This refreshing drink is a hit turned into Popsicles.*

2 cups (500 ml) ginger-oatstraw tea

2 cups (500 ml) raspberry juice

## HERBAL LEMONADE

*We make herbal lemonade for most every family gathering. No one misses the sodas; this lemonade is a festive and satisfying treat that is good for you.*

2 cups (500 ml) herbal tea

½ cup (185 ml) honey

½ cup (125 ml) fresh lemon juice

Lemon slices for garnish

> Put 1 cup (250 ml) of the tea and the honey into a saucepan over low heat. Stir until the honey liquefies and blends into the tea. Pour the tea-honey mixture into a pitcher and add the remaining 1 cup (250 ml) of the tea and the fresh lemon juice. Chill and serve garnished with fresh lemon slices.

## LEMON VERBENA LEMONADE

*The aromatic, floral explosion of lemon verbena in your lemonade makes a first-rate drink for all special occasions.*

4 cups (1 L) lemon verbena tea

1 cup (250 ml) fresh lemon juice

1 cup (370 ml) honey

## OATSTRAW BREEZE

*This makes a very satisfying summer tea. All the ingredients nourish the nervous system and help to invite a calmness into the busy schedule of summer.*

2 cups (500 ml) oatstraw-lavender tea

2 tablespoons (30 ml) rose water

¼ cup (93 ml) rose petal honey

Seasonal fruit for garnish

## PARADISE POTION

*Once you bring this delightful drink to a party, people start requesting that you bring drinks instead of food to potlucks!*

2 cups (500 ml) blush wine

2 cups (500 ml) lavender or lemon verbena tea

½ cup (250 ml) frozen lemonade concentrate

¼ cup (60 ml) rose water

½ cup (125 ml) orange juice

2 cups (500 ml) carbonated water

Thinly sliced strawberries

Thinly sliced oranges

Thinly sliced limes

Stir together all the liquid ingredients in a punch bowl and float the fruit slices in the bowl.

## PARTY PUNCH

*This delightful drink is a holiday favorite. It is easy to throw together, and everyone loves it. I make it for weddings and large celebrations. Serve it in a punch bowl.*

4 cups (1 L) lemon verbena–rose petal tea

4 cups (1 L) berry juice

Fresh berries for garnish

Rose petals for garnish

## PEPPERMINT-LAVENDER LEMONADE

*When we have parties, we fill a 5-gallon (20-L) Igloo water dispenser with peppermint-lavender lemonade. Everyone loves it, and it costs a fraction of what it would cost to supply the masses with sodas or packaged drinks.*

2 cups (500 ml) lavender and peppermint tea

½ cup (125 ml) fresh lemon juice

½ cup (185 ml) honey

Peppermint sprigs for garnish

Lemon slices for garnish

## RASPBERRY-ROSE GERANIUM JUICE

1 cup (125 g) raspberries

1 cup (250 ml) rose geranium tea

1 cup (250 ml) berry juice

¼ cup (18 g) fresh rose geranium

¼ cup (24 g) fresh lemon balm

¼ teaspoon (¼ g) powdered allspice

3 tablespoons (70 ml) honey (or to taste)

> Put all ingredients except for the honey into the blender and blend well. Pour the herbed fruit purée through a piece of muslin into a glass pitcher and squeeze out all of the juice. Discard the fruit. Add honey.

## ROSE COOLER

*I am always trying to find ways to interest people in using herbs. This lively cocktail has done the job of just that. Herbal teas can elevate just about any drink you can imagine.*

1 cup (250 ml) rose petal–rose hip tea

1 cup (250 ml) organic berry juice

2 cups (500 ml) carbonated water

1 cup (250 ml) white wine

Rose petals for garnish

Lime slices for garnish

> Combine all liquid ingredients in a pitcher; add rose petals and lime slices for garnish; serve chilled.

## SUMMER HERBAL ICED TEA

*This is the perfect tea to refresh and revitalize. It helps you to avoid an afternoon energy crash and enlivens the mind.*

4 cups (1 L) orange peel–peppermint tea

Honey to taste

Fresh lemon juice to taste

## SUMMER SPARKLE

¼ cup Ginger Honey (page 165)

4 cups (1 L) peppermint–lemon balm tea

½ cup (125 ml) orange juice concentrate or lemon juice concentrate

Lemon balm sprigs for garnish

> Warm the honey, stir it into the tea, add the juice concentrate, and then chill. Garnish with lemon balm sprigs.

## VITAMIN C THIRST QUENCHER

2 cups (500 ml) chamomile–rose hip tea

2 tablespoons (30 ml) berry juice concentrate

1 tablespoon (15 ml) fresh lime juice

**WARM DRINKS**

## ASTRAGALUS AND APPLE JUICE

*Astragalus helps us to prepare for the coming cold and flu season, which makes it a perfect ingredient for this favorite fall treat when the apples are ripe. Autumn weather alternates between hot and cold, so sip this drink slightly chilled on warmer days, or drink it hot in a mug by the fire when the weather is cold.*

2 cups (500 ml) astragalus tea

1½ (375 ml) cups apple juice

Pinch of cinnamon

Pinch of allspice

## AUTUMN SPICE

*Adding this robust blend of herbs to apple cider makes a delicious, hearty drink.*

4 cups (1 L) orange, cinnamon, and ginger tea

3 cups (750 ml) apple cider

## COLD CARE TEA

*This is a simple and delicious tea that will chase away a cold.*

2 cups (500 ml) rose hip–elderberry tea

1 teaspoon (8 ml) lavender honey

## DANDELION MOCHA

*For years I have recommended this recipe in my herbal consultation practice as a substitute for coffee drinks. I have witnessed hundreds of people wean themselves off their coffee addictions with the help of roasted dandelion drinks.*

3 cups (750 ml) water

3 tablespoons (45 g) roasted dandelion root

1 tablespoon (8 g) raw cocoa nibs

½ cup (125 ml) raw milk or almond milk

½ teaspoon (1 g) powdered cinnamon

½ teaspoon (3 ml) vanilla extract/essence

2 tablespoons (30 ml) barley malt syrup/essence

1 tablespoon (22 ml) maple syrup (if desired, for more sweetness)

Dash of powdered clove

Dash of powdered nutmeg

> Make a tea from the water, dandelion root, and cocoa nibs. Let steep for 30 minutes. Strain the tea, add the remaining ingredients, and reheat.

 ## ENERGIZER BREW

*This hearty drink is a choice blend for promoting energy and vitality.*

2 cups astragalus and ginger tea

2 tablespoons Chai Honey (page 162)

 ## GINGER COLD BUSTER

*Drink this hot at the very first sign of a cold. Rest after you drink a cup; when you wake up, the cold will have disappeared.*

1 cup (250 ml) ginger tea

2 tablespoons (45 ml) Cinnamon-Ginger Honey (pages 162–163)

1 to 2 tablespoons (15 to 30 ml) fresh lemon juice

## HERBAL HONEY TEA

*A simple way to make tea is to just add hot water to an already made herbal honey.*

1 teaspoon to 1 tablespoon (8 to 23 ml) of herbal honey (see chapter 6)

1 cup (250 ml) hot water

> Just add the honey to hot water, stir until the honey is thoroughly mixed into the water, and drink.

## HERBED CHAI

*Transform this choice hot beverage into a nice latte-type drink by using a hand immersion blender to blend the milk into the tea until foamy.*

2 cups (500 ml) water

2 tablespoons (45 ml) Chai Honey (page 162)

¼ cup (60 ml) raw milk or almond milk

Dash of powdered cardamom

## IMMUNE JUICE

*This fusion of herbs, juice, and honey makes an exceptionally pleasant drink for building immunity.*

2 cups (500 ml) elderberry–astragalus tea

1 cup (150 ml) pomegranate juice

1 teaspoon (8 ml) Ginger Honey (page 165)

Cinnamon stick for garnish

## LONGEVITY ELIXIR

*This is the perfect after-dinner tea on a cold night.*

2 cups (500 ml) fennel, chamomile, and coriander tea

1 teaspoon (8 ml) nutmeg honey

## MULLED CIDER

*People feel welcomed by the warming, spicy smell of these herbs infusing in the kitchen.*

4 quarts (4 L) apple cider

5 cinnamon sticks

5 astragalus sticks

2 tablespoons (5 g) allspice berries

1 teaspoon (4 g) powdered clove

1 teaspoon (2 g) powdered nutmeg

Peel from one orange

Pour the cider into a large pot over low heat. Put the herbs into a piece of muslin. You can purchase empty, premade muslin pouches, or just make your own, tying the fabric closed with a piece of string. Put the bag full of herbs into the apple cider and let them infuse for one hour before drinking. Keep the cider warm on the lowest stove setting and leave the bag of herbs in the pot until the cider is finished.

## REJUVENATION TEA

*This is a thick and sweet tea that tastes so yummy, it takes the place of dessert.*

2 cups (500 ml) fennel, orange peel, and coriander tea

1 cup (250 ml) almond milk

4 dates, pitted

¼ teaspoon (½ g) powdered cinnamon

Pinch of nutmeg

Add all ingredients to the blender and blend until the dates are smooth. Pour the mixture into a pot on low heat for a few minutes and serve warm.

## SOOTHE AND IMPROVE TEA

2 cups (250 ml) ginger, burdock, and dandelion root tea

1 teaspoon (8 ml) cardamom honey

## SPICED WINE

*This is a favorite drink at all our winter season celebrations.*

1 bottle of red wine

1 teaspoon (4 g) juniper berries

1 teaspoon (2 g) whole fennel seeds

¼ teaspoon (1 g) minced fresh ginger

1 whole clove

In a large pot over low heat, combine all the ingredients. Bring to a simmer, turn the heat to the lowest setting, and serve warm.

## WARMING WINTER BREW

*This is a warm, full-bodied tea that has a revitalizing effect on a cold winter day.*

1 cup (250 ml) ginger-cinnamon tea

1 teaspoon (7 ml) molasses/treacle

1 teaspoon (8 ml) star anise honey

# Herbal Smoothies

I was raised on the western edge of the Sacramento Valley. I still live here, and I love it; I love the hills, the oak trees, and the sweltering summer heat. Summer temperatures are often over 100°F/38°C for weeks. Dipping into water and drinking chilled drinks is a necessity. Each day you search for something to extinguish the insatiable thirst that comes with the heat that doesn't seem to ever let up. The pursuit for the ultimate thirst quencher is a way of life in hot climates.

Living here, one understands the true meaning of refreshment. The heat is sometimes relentless, and the perfect beverage truly does refresh and rejuvenate. When someone walks in the door, you offer them something to drink. I enjoy having special drinks in the summer—something a little extra, more than ice water or bottled juice. I grew up with my grandparents always having a pitcher full of chilled, sugar-loaded Lipton iced tea in the refrigerator. That was the hospitality beverage of choice served during a time when it was customary for neighbors and friends to stop by for a chat or morning coffee or tea.

We live in the land of plenty when it comes to the fruit harvest. Each season brings on a new delicacy, one fruit after another. What a celebration when the cherries first come, but it isn't so difficult to say goodbye to them, because here come the apricots, then the peaches and pears and on and on. The smoothies just evolve through the summer with each ripening fruit. Get into the habit of making an herbal tea at night before you go to bed. In the morning the tea is ready to use as the chief ingredient for the soothing, therapeutic drink that everyone will be asking for.

# GETTING STARTED

**SUPPLIES**

blender

**INGREDIENTS**

Fresh and dried herbs for making tea

> Once you get in the habit of making daily herbal teas, adding tea to your smoothies is easy. The teas contribute a kaleidoscope of nutrients and flavor that turns smoothie-making into an altogether different experience than just blending fruit.

Sprigs of fresh herbs for adding to smoothies

> Blend sprigs of fresh herbs into smoothies, such as basil, cilantro, dandelion leaves, lemon balm, lemon verbena, peppermint, rosemary, rose geranium, and rose petals. Herbal smoothies are a great place to sneak more leafy greens into your diet. Even if you are making a summer treat with bananas and strawberries, you can add a handful of fresh parsley or peppermint.

Fresh or frozen fruit

> Each fruit has a different consistency and flavor that will dictate what else goes into the smoothie. Fresh fruits like banana, mango, apple, pineapple, and kiwi don't usually need a sweetener, whereas strawberry, pomegranate, blueberry, and blackberry smoothies may require a little honey. Some berries are mild and sweet, like mulberries, and some berries are astringent and bitter, like raspberries. The bitter berries may take more sweetener than other fruits, depending on your taste.
>
> If you want to add honey or syrup, it is easier to blend it into the tea before the fruit is added. Frozen fruit will give your smoothie a cold, crunchy texture without needing ice.

Ice

> If you use frozen fruit in your smoothie, there is no need for ice.

Whole plain yogurt

> Avoid low-fat yogurt; instead use organic yogurt made from whole milk.

### Kefir

A little kefir in your smoothie adds flavor and is full of beneficial bacteria that builds strong digestion.

### Herbed or fruited vinegar

See chapter 7 for vinegar recipes.

### Fermented vegetable juice

I am always looking for ways to sneak more fermented foods into our diet. Fermented foods are a very important staple for helping to replenish the beneficial bacteria in the gut. Healthy beneficial bacteria increase our ability to digest our food, and they also enhance the immune system. If you have sauerkraut in the refrigerator, you can pour a little of the juice into smoothies.

### Nut milk

Almond milk is a wonderful addition to your smoothies and is easily made at home. Almonds, like most nuts, need to be soaked overnight to remove the enzyme inhibitors.

1. Soak 1 cup (170 g) of organic almonds overnight in 2 cups (500 ml) of water.
2. Pour off the soaking water and rinse the almonds in a colander.
3. Put the soaked almonds and 2 cups (500 ml) of fresh water in the blender, and blend until creamy.
4. For sweet almond milk, add three pitted dates and blend.
5. You can either leave the almond pulp in the liquid or strain it out. I leave it in, but some people complain about the small pieces in the milk. To strain out the pulp, let the mixture sit for a few minutes, and then pour the milk through muslin into a clean jar or container. When all the liquid is poured out of the blender, squeeze the cloth until all the milk is drained. The remaining almond pulp can be stored for a couple of days in the refrigerator and is delicious in pancakes and baked or dehydrated cookies/biscuits.
6. Store the almond milk in a sealed container in the refrigerator for up to four days.

# MAKING HERBAL SMOOTHIES

## METHOD

1. Make a tea with fresh or dried herbs; use a single herb tea or a tea blend.

2. Strain herbs from the tea.

3. Put tea in the blender. If you would like to add honey to sweeten your smoothie, add honey to the blender before adding fresh or frozen fruit, and blend to mix with the tea.

4. Add chopped fresh fruit or frozen fruit to the blender and blend well.

5. Add sprigs of fresh herbs and blend.

6. Add other ingredients as desired: yogurt, kefir, nut milk, a splash of herbal vinegar or sauerkraut juice, powdered seaweed, herbed honey, more fresh green herbs, or herbal sprinkles.

## STORAGE

Drink herbal smoothies right away or store them in the refrigerator overnight. You can also freeze smoothies for a couple months in Mason jars or put them in Popsicle molds and make summer frozen pops. When freezing smoothies in a Mason jar, be sure to fill the jar only halfway full with the smoothie. If you fill the jar all the way up it, the expansion that takes place with freezing can cause the jar to explode.

# RECISPES

The smoothie recipes that follow are designed to be blended in the blender. They are summer drinks; it isn't good to drink ice-cold drinks in the winter. I put much less ice in our smoothies than you would find in a smoothie you purchased at the juice bar. Too much ice is hard on the stomach, so use just enough ice or frozen fruit to give your smoothie the thick, crunchy texture you are looking for. Drink these smoothies chilled, but not too cold. Frozen drinks hinder digestion and can cause mucus. Drink smoothies in the middle of the day, not at night when your digestion slows. If you have mucus or allergies, refrain from cold smoothies altogether. Avoid the mistake of carrying on with your summer smoothie habit into the fall. Once the weather starts cooling down, transition into drinking beverages that are room temperature or warm.

Kids love making smoothies, so teach them how to make their own summer drinks. Have fun experimenting with what you have on hand. Get in the habit of making herbal smoothies as a summer treat to replace all the high-fructose corn syrup ice pops, snow cones, and the endless onslaught of insulting snacks marketed to children.

## BERRY BLAST

*This is a satisfying summer smoothie that supports cardiovascular health and keeps you cool and refreshed on a sweltering summer day.*

1 cup (250 ml) rose petal–hawthorn berry tea

2 tablespoons (44 ml) maple syrup

1 cup (125 g) frozen berries

2 tablespoons (30 ml) rose water

1 teaspoon (5 ml) Fruited Vinegar (pages 179–180)

1 teaspoon (5 ml) Vanilla Cordial (page 203)

Handful of fresh rose petals

Add tea and maple syrup to blender and blend. Add the remaining ingredients and blend until the frozen berries are completely mixed into the liquid.

## BERRY-MINT FIZZ

*See chapter 6 for options on some herbal honeys.*

1 cup (250 ml) peppermint tea

3 tablespoons (70 ml) herbal honey

1 cup (125 g) frozen berries

2 tablespoons (30 ml) fresh lime juice

1 pinch of stevia powder

Handful of fresh peppermint

1 cup (250 ml) carbonated water (optional)

> Add tea and honey to blender and blend until mixed. Add the berries, lime juice, stevia powder, and peppermint and blend until evenly mixed. Stir in carbonated water, if using, just before serving.

## FEELIN' GROOVY

*I love peach season! This smoothie is one we drink quite often, but feel free to experiment with other teas to complement your peaches.*

1 cup (250 ml) rose geranium tea

2 cups (370 g) fresh peach slices (about 1½ medium peaches)

½ vanilla bean/pod, chopped

⅛ teaspoon (½ ml) stevia extract/essence

1 tablespoon (15 ml) Fruited Vinegar (pages 179–180)

¼ teaspoon (½ g) powdered cardamom

½ to 1 cup (63 to 125 g) crushed ice

## FIVE-FLOWER FUSION

*Blend these floral ingredients together and enjoy their health-giving properties.*

3 cups (750 ml) calendula, chamomile, elder flower, lavender, and rose petal tea

¼ cup (94 ml) rose petal honey

½ cup (63 g) crushed ice

⅛ cup (6 g) fresh rose petals

## GARDEN SMOOTHIE

*I love going into the garden and picking a handful of vibrant, edible herbs and flowers and putting them into my smoothie. This recipes calls for a handful of peppermint, but I often also pick parsley or calendula for this smoothie.*

1 cup (250 ml) peppermint, rosemary, and rose petal tea

1 cup (250 ml) pear juice

2 tablespoons (30 ml) pomegranate concentrate

Handful of fresh peppermint

½ cup (63 g) ice

## GO GREEN

*Drinking a glass full of greens is a great pick-me-up. Infuse yourself with the vitamins and chlorophyll that the herbs offer, and watch your energy soar.*

1 to 2 cups (250 to 500 ml) herbal tea

1 cup (250 ml) almond milk

1 fresh apple

½ banana

½ cup (15 g) fresh parsley

½ cup (15 g) fresh cilantro

½ cup (36 g) fresh dandelion leaf

1 teaspoon (1 g) powdered seaweed

1 tablespoon (5 to 8 g) herb sprinkle

## KIWI TWIST

*A splash of Fruited Vinegar (pages 179–180) or Lavender-Rosemary Vinegar (page 183) adds a zest of lively flavor to this smoothie.*

1 cup (250 ml) rose geranium tea

1½ cups (185 g) fresh kiwi slices

1 teaspoon (8 ml) honey

1 tablespoon (15 ml) herbed vinegar

½ cup (63 g) crushed ice

## LEMON VERBENA NECTAR

*My five-year-old son created this recipe; he is definitely a smoothie kid. I have a lazy Susan with several herbal honeys and herbal sprinkles sitting by the blender. He uses whatever tea I have leftover from the morning, a mix-and-match of honey and sprinkles, and his favorite fruit, blueberries. He calls all of the smoothies "green drinks" even though this one is blue.*

1 cup (250 ml) lemon verbena tea

1 tablespoon (23 ml) Ginger Honey (page 165)

1 cup (125 g) frozen blueberries

Handful of fresh lemon balm

> Add tea and honey to blender and blend until mixed well. Add the frozen berries and lemon balm and blend until evenly mixed.

## ROSE JULEP

1 cup (250 ml) rose petal tea

4 teaspoons (20 ml) fresh lemon juice

2 tablespoons (30 ml) cup rose water

3 tablespoons (70 ml) rose hip honey

Handful of fresh rose petals

½ cup (63 g) crushed ice

Lime slices for garnish

## SPICED ROSE HIP SLUSH

*Take your smoothies to another level by adding herb-infused honey. Plain honey tastes just fine, but try your hand at making a few herbal honeys and see what it does for your drinks! See chapter 6 for instructions and recipes for herbal honey.*

1½ cups (375 ml) rose hip–cinnamon tea

1 tablespoon (23 ml) honey infused with orange peel, star anise, ginger, and clove

1 cup (125 g) fresh blackberries

Sprig of fresh peppermint

½ cup (63 g) crushed ice

> Add tea and honey to blender and blend until mixed well. Add the fresh berries, peppermint, and ice and blend until evenly mixed.

##  STRAWBERRY CRUSH

*The first strawberries are a sure sign that winter is over. The salutation to spring is expressed in the exuberance in which strawberries are welcomed into our meals. If you avoid fruits that are not in season and don't eat strawberries all year long, then it really is festival time when the strawberries arrive. It always feels like a celebration when we get to add straw-berries to our drinks. This drink is one of our favorites. I love that we receive the benefits of nutrient-rich herbs in something that tastes like dessert!*

1 cup (250 ml) oatstraw-calendula tea

1 tablespoon (22 ml) maple syrup

1 cup (125 g) fresh strawberries

1 banana

¼ cup (63 g) yogurt

½ cup (63 g) crushed ice

Pinch of cardamom

##  SUMMER PEACH

1 cup (250 ml) lavender tea

2 tablespoons (45 ml) rose hip honey

2 cups (370 g) fresh peach slices (about 1½ medium peaches)

Dash of powdered clove

2 sprigs of fresh peppermint

Small handful of ice

## TROPICAL CREAM

1 cup (250 ml) ginger-lavender tea

1½ cups (93 g) chopped fresh pineapple

½ cup (125 ml) coconut milk

1 tablespoon (15 ml) coconut oil

8 dates, pitted

¼ teaspoon (½ g) cardamom

⅛ teaspoon (¼ g) powdered nutmeg

Handful of fresh lemon balm

½ cup (63 g) crushed ice

## WATERMELON-MINT FRAPPE

*This is an indispensable summer drink when the days are just too hot.*

1 cup (250 ml) peppermint tea

3 to 4 cups (555 to 740 g) watermelon cubes

Sprig of fresh rose geranium

1 cup (125 g) crushed ice

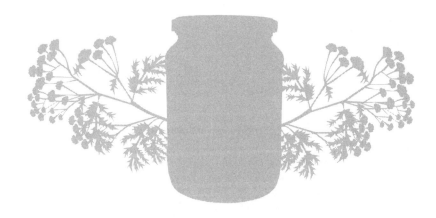

# CHAPTER 6

# Herbal Honey

Honey is another ingredient that everyone has in their cupboard. How do you use honey in your kitchen? In whatever way you eat or drink honey, you can enhance its medicinal qualities by adding herbs to it. Herbal honeys are easy to make and a great way to get herbs into your diet. In almost any capacity that you use honey, an herbal honey can be the substitute. Add herbal honey to your warm cereal, put it on breakfast toast and waffles, use it instead of jam, or bake it into a dessert. Your peanut butter and honey sandwich will never be the same. Use it as syrup and put it in marinades, salad dressings or sauces for main dishes and mix it into tea. We even put honey on our popcorn! Whether you use it in your breakfast foods or to sweeten your beverages, you are going to love the flavors that unfold when you fortify your honey with herbs.

# GETTING STARTED

**SUPPLIES**

clean, sterilized jar

double boiler

**INGREDIENTS**

Honey

Making herbal honey is easy, and everyone loves the added surprise of herbs and dried fruit to spice things up a bit. The best honey to use is one that is local to where you live. Try to find a beekeeper in your area that sells honey, and purchase honey that is raw and has not been heated. Raw honey is full of healing enzymes that are destroyed in the heating process. Some of the honey available in stores is processed and heated, and many commercial honeys are not labeled with the information of whether they are cooked or not. When you buy honey from someone local, you can ask them about their processing methods and whether they heat the honey. Honey is antibacterial and antioxidant. Adding honey to food and drinks enhances the absorption of nutrients and helps to deliver the medicinal qualities of herbs deeper in to the body. Give thanks to the bees!

Dried fruit

The fruit for these recipes needs to be dried and chopped into small pieces. Dried peaches, apricots, figs, cherries, currants, pears, and raisins are my favorite dried fruits to add to honey. Dried fruit infuses an extra bounty of vitamins and flavor to your herbal honeys.

Powdered herbs

Herbs need to be dried and finely powdered before being mixed into honey. Many herbs can be powdered in your kitchen using a blender or coffee grinder. Some herbs are too fluffy or too woody and need to be powdered with commercial-grade equipment in order to break them down sufficiently. It is easy enough to purchase powdered herbs.

# MAKING HERBAL HONEY

## PROPORTIONS

¼ to ½ cup (4 to 48 g) of dried herbs to 1 cup (370 ml) of honey

½ to ¾ cup (93 to 139 g) of dried fruit to 1 cup (370 ml) of honey

For culinary uses, ¼ cup (4 to 24 g) of dried herbs is usually enough for 1 cup (370 ml) of honey. If you are making herbed honey for more therapeutic purposes or to add to medicinal teas, then you can experiment with adding up to ½ cup (metric) of dried herbs per one cup of honey. These proportions are a general guideline. As with all of the recipes, I encourage you to get a feel for what you are doing and then experiment to find out what you like best.

### METHOD #1: HONEY WITH POWDERED HERBS

Over the years, I have made many honeys where the herbs were just chopped or grated and not powdered. I found that the herbs really do need to be finely powdered for a pleasant honey-eating experience! When I first tried making herbal honey, I found a recipe that talked about straining the herbs from the honey. Ha. That was a good joke. It takes forever and is not something that you are inspired to do twice. If you really want the herbs removed from your honey, then don't powder them. Leave the herbs whole during the steeping process. If you warm the honey, then straining the herbs out is a little easier.

1 cup (370 ml) honey

¼ to ½ cup (24 to 48 g) powdered herbs

1. Put honey into a sterilized jar.
2. Put the jar into a double boiler over low heat.
3. Gently heat for fifteen minutes, or until it is warm. Do not boil or overheat the honey, just warm it up until the herbs can be easily mixed in.
4. Stir the herbs into the honey while it is still warm.
5. Remove jar of honey from double boiler and let cool.

6. Store the honey in a cabinet for two weeks before eating.

7. Occasionally stir the contents, mixing herbs thoroughly into the honey.

8. Just leave the herbs in the honey as you use it. There is no need to strain the herbs out at any point.

## METHOD #2: HONEY WITH DRIED FRUIT

If you are adding only fruit to the honey, there is no need to heat it. If you decide to add herbs as well, simply warm the honey and herbs as described in Method #1, remove from the heat, and proceed with step 1 below.

1 cup honey
½ to ¾ cup (93 to 139 g) dried, chopped fruit

1. Add dried, chopped fruit to the honey and mix well.

2. Let fruited honey steep for two weeks before eating.

3. Do not strain the fruit from the honey; eat it right along with the honey.

## STORAGE

Herbal honeys are very stable. We keep several herbal honeys in the pantry and a few can be found on the kitchen table, so they are conveniently added to breakfast. Because the honeys are made with all dried ingredients, they can easily last for one year outside of the refrigerator. Sometimes the herbs settle a little and the honey needs a good stirring.

# RECITES

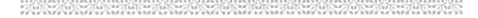

Following are some of my favorite herbal honey recipes, but be sure to look around and see what ingredients are local and seasonal and in abundance in your cupboard.

## APRICOT-LAVENDER HONEY

*One summer, I had a bumper crop of apricots and lavender flowers and decided to preserve them into honey. I made so much that there was enough to last through the winter, so it naturally ended up as a Christmas present for friends and family. It was a hit, everyone loved it, and I took care of everyone on my Christmas list in one afternoon!*

1 cup (370 ml) honey

¾ cup (139 g) finely chopped dried apricots

2 tablespoons (12 g) powdered lavender

¼ teaspoon (½ g) powdered nutmeg

## BARBECUE HONEY GLAZE

*Spread this on chicken, pork chops, or skewered veggies. The herbs help to tenderize and add a delicious flavor.*

1 cup (370 ml) honey

2 tablespoons (12 g) powdered ginger

1 tablespoon (6 g) powdered rosemary

2 teaspoons (3 g) powdered thyme

## BODY GLOW HONEY

*Get wet, scrub this all over, and let it soak into your skin for about 15 minutes. Shower off and glow!*

1 cup (370 ml) honey

2 tablespoons (12 g) powdered lemon balm

2 tablespoons (12 g) powdered chamomile

1 tablespoon (6 g) powdered lavender

1 tablespoon (6 g) powdered mugwort

1 teaspoon (2 g) powdered rosemary

 ## CHAI HONEY

*Make a delicious cup of chai by adding 1 tablespoon (23 ml) of Chai Honey to ¾ cup (180 ml) water and ¼ cup (60 ml) raw milk or almond milk. Herbal chai is a champion afternoon pick-me-up and substitute for coffee. Chai Honey is a great traveling companion. Put your Chai Honey in a jar when you travel and just add it to hot water.*

2 cups (740 ml) honey

3 tablespoons (21 g) powdered cinnamon

2 tablespoons (12 g) powdered coriander

1½ teaspoons (3 g) powdered clove

1½ teaspoons (3 g) powdered cardamom

1 teaspoon (2 g) powdered ginger

1 teaspoon (2 g) powdered black pepper

 ## CINNAMON HONEY

*This honey turns toast into a yummy treat and livens up pancakes, waffles, and all warm breakfast cereals. If you are catching a cold, make a tea with just Cinnamon Honey, and it will help to send your cold on its way. To make the tea, put 1 tablespoon (23 ml) of Cinnamon Honey into 1 cup (250 ml) of hot water and let it cool a bit before drinking. Drink two or three servings a day at the onset of a cold.*

1 cup (370 ml) honey

3 tablespoons (21 g) powdered cinnamon

1 teaspoon (1 g) powdered allspice

 ## CINNAMON-GINGER HONEY

*We keep this honey on our kitchen table and put it on morning quinoa. It also makes a delicious digestive tea or flavoring for pancake batter and muffins. Keep it on the table in the winter and use it to keep away colds. Spreading Cinnamon-Ginger Honey on your*

*morning toast can warm you up on a winter morning, reduce your susceptibility to a cold,
and stimulate digestion.*

1 cup (370 ml) honey

2 tablespoons (14 g) powdered cinnamon

1 tablespoon (6 g) powdered ginger

## COUGH-EASE HONEY

*Make a tea with this honey for wet coughs with excess mucus.*

1 cup (370 ml) honey

2 tablespoons (6 g) powdered fennel seed

1 teaspoon (2 g) powdered star anise

¾ teaspoon (1½ g) powdered black pepper

½ teaspoon (½ g) powdered ginger

## CURRIED HONEY

*If you like curry, this is an exemplary honey for cooking. Put 3 tablespoons on a chicken
before baking, or mix it with baked vegetables. The results are unbelievably scrumptious.*

2 cups (740 ml) honey

2 tablespoons (12 g) powdered coriander

1 tablespoon (6 g) powdered cumin

1 tablespoon (6 g) powdered turmeric

2 teaspoons (6 g) powdered mustard seed

2 teaspoons (2 g) powdered fennel seed

½ teaspoon (1 g) powdered cinnamon

½ teaspoon (1 g) powdered ginger

¼ teaspoon (½ g) powdered clove

## DIGESTIVE AID SPICE HONEY

*For a wonderful tea to sip after a substantial meal, add 1 teaspoon (8 ml) of this honey to
a cup of warm water and stir. If your lunch or dinner makes you sleepy, it is because your
energy is going to your digestive tract to help you to process your food. Let your herbal honey*

*help you to digest: drink some of this tea, and you can avoid the afternoon slump that often accompanies a hearty meal.*

1 cup (370 ml) honey

2 tablespoons (12 g) powdered orange peel

1 tablespoon (6 g) powdered dandelion root

1 teaspoon (2 g) powdered ginger

½ teaspoon (1 g) powdered star anise

½ teaspoon (1 g) powdered clove

## FLEXIBILITY HONEY

*All of the herbs in this honey help to reduce inflammation and increase circulation throughout the body. Adding turmeric and ginger to your diet helps with arthritic complaints. You can also warm this honey up and scrub it on your feet. Leave it on for ten minutes and wash off with warm water. The honey foot rub will warm your body and increase circulation.*

2 cups (740 ml) honey

1 tablespoon (6 g) powdered turmeric

1 teaspoon (2 g) powdered ginger

1 teaspoon (2 g) powdered juniper berry

½ teaspoon (1 g) powdered cardamom

## FRUITED HONEY

*To create an all-purpose spread, blend this honey in a food processor with cream cheese.*

1½ cups (555 ml) honey

1 cup (185 g) finely chopped dried pears

¼ cup (47 g) chopped raisins

2 tablespoons (12 g) powdered orange peel

1 teaspoon (2 g) powdered rose hips

¼ teaspoon (½ g) powdered cardamom

½ teaspoon (½ g) powdered allspice

½ vanilla bean/pod, finely chopped

## GINGER HONEY

*I make this honey specifically for adding to lemonade. There are lots of lemon trees in our neighborhood. We juice the lemons, add Ginger Honey, and make a lemonade that can be served hot or cold.*

1 cup (370 ml) honey

¼ cup (24 g) powdered ginger

## GINGER-FIG HONEY

*Spread cream cheese or goat cheese on crackers and drizzle with this honey for the perfect party hors d'oeuvre.*

1 cup (370 ml) honey

1½ cups (278 g) finely chopped dried fig

¾ teaspoon (1½ g) powdered ginger

¼ teaspoon (½ g) powdered star anise

¼ teaspoon (½ g) nutmeg

## HAPPY TUMMY HONEY

*Make a cup of Happy Tummy Honey tea when you have an upset stomach. Add 1 teaspoon (8 ml) to 1 tablespoon (23 ml) of Happy Tummy Honey to 1 cup (250 ml) hot water and mix well.*

1 cup (370 ml) honey

2 tablespoons (12 g) powdered fennel seed

2 tablespoons (12 g) powdered coriander

1 teaspoon (1 g) powdered cumin

## HEART TONIC HONEY

*This honey is a cardiovascular tonic that lends itself well to morning foods. We also like to warm it up and add it to yogurt. Yum.*

1 cup (370 ml) honey

2 tablespoons (12 g) powdered hawthorn berry

1 tablespoon (6 g) powdered rose hips

1 teaspoon (2 g) powdered cinnamon

½ teaspoon (1 g) powdered ginger

## HONEY FACIAL MASK

*Honey is a gentle astringent and anti–inflammatory for facial tissue. It tightens up tired skin and reduces puffiness and redness. Apply a warm washcloth to your face for several minutes to soften the skin, then apply this Honey Facial Mask to the face and leave on for ten minutes. Rinse off with warm water. This honey is also a good disinfecting and healing application for superficial wounds.*

1 cup (370 ml) honey

¼ cup (24 g) powdered chamomile

¼ cup (24 g) powdered elder flower

## HONEY SPREAD

*Drizzle this honey over baked Brie or use it as a spread for cheese and crackers/savory biscuits.*

1 cup (370 ml) honey

1 cup (180 g) finely chopped crystallized ginger

1 cup (125 g) finely chopped cranberries

1 tablespoon (6 g) powdered orange peel

1 tablespoon (6 g) powdered rose hips

## LAVENDER-ORANGE HONEY

*This is an exquisite honey mixed into breakfast foods or added to marinades.*

1 cup (370 ml) honey

¾ cup (139 g) finely chopped dates

1 tablespoon (6 g) powdered lavender

1 tablespoon (6 g) powdered orange peel

1 teaspoon (2 g) powdered lemon verbena

## MORNING WARMTH HONEY

*This makes a wonderful tea when you have a hard time getting going in the morning. Put 1 teaspoon (8 ml) of Morning Warmth Honey into 1 cup (250 ml) of hot water. You can also use this honey to flavor and sweeten other warm morning drinks.*

1 cup (370 ml) honey

2 tablespoons (14 g) powdered cinnamon

2 teaspoons (4 g) powdered ginger

1 teaspoon (2 g) powdered fennel seed

1 teaspoon (2 g) powdered astragalus

¼ teaspoon (½ g) powdered cardamom

## POPCORN HONEY

*We are such "herbies" that we even add herbal mixtures to our popcorn!*

1 cup (370 ml) honey

2 teaspoons (4 g) powdered garlic

½ teaspoon (1 g) powdered ginger

Dash of powdered cayenne

## POULTRY GLAZE HONEY

1 cup (370 ml) honey

2 tablespoons (12 g) powdered coriander

2 teaspoons (4 g) powdered paprika

1 teaspoon (2 g) powdered cumin

1 teaspoon (2 g) powdered turmeric

1 teaspoon (1 g) powdered thyme

1 teaspoon (2 g) powdered black pepper

½ teaspoon (1 g) powdered clove

½ teaspoon (1 g) powdered celery seed

## RESPIRATORY RELIEF HONEY

*Make up a batch of this honey in the fall to use all winter long. The minute your throat starts to feel scratchy, just suck on a small spoonful of Respiratory Relief Honey. It will soothe and disinfect your throat, prevent the sore throat from getting worse, and generally keep colds at bay.*

1½ cups (555 ml) honey

3 tablespoons (18 g) powdered fennel seed

2 teaspoons (4 g) powdered juniper berry

2 teaspoons (4 g) powdered ginger

1 teaspoon (2 g) powdered horseradish

1 teaspoon (2 g) powdered garlic

## ROSE DELIGHT HONEY

*This honey makes a delicious tea to help prevent colds and soothe sore throats. I use it in cakes instead of sugar, and my son eats it on his French toast and muffins. What you don't eat for breakfast can be applied as a facial mask to revive your skin and give you a glowing complexion.*

1 cup (370 ml) honey

3 tablespoons (18 g) powdered rose hips

2 tablespoons (12 g) powdered rose petals

## ROSEMARY HONEY

*This is a good honey to use in salad dressings or as a hair conditioner. Yes, a hair conditioner! If you want to have gorgeous, shining hair, simply get your hair wet and smother your head with honey. Leave the honey on for about one hour, rinse it off, then wash your hair as you normally would. Try it.*

1 cup (370 ml) honey

¼ cup (24 g) powdered rosemary

## SLEEPY TIME HONEY

*Make a tea with this honey to help clean out the day and pave the way for a good night's sleep.*

1 cup (370 ml) honey

2 tablespoons (12 g) powdered lavender

2 tablespoons (12 g) powdered chamomile

1 teaspoon (2 g) powdered lemon balm

½ teaspoon (1 g) powdered nutmeg

## SPICED HONEY

*This is a handy marinade honey to have around. It helps with digestion, calms the nerves, uplifts the spirit, and chases colds away.*

1 cup (370 ml) honey

2 tablespoons (12 g) powdered lavender

1 tablespoon (6 g) powdered rosemary

1 tablespoon (6 g) powdered fennel seed

½ teaspoon (1 g) powdered cinnamon

½ teaspoon (1 g) powdered nutmeg

## TAMARI HONEY MARINADE

*This is a staple ingredient in my refrigerator. It turns any stir-fry into an epicurean delight.*

¼ cup (60 ml) tamari

¼ cup (93 ml) Ginger Honey (page 165)

1 garlic clove, minced

> Mix ingredients and let sit for a couple of hours before using. This sauce is good for about two weeks or more stored in the refrigerator.

## TURMERIC HONEY

*There is more turmeric in this honey than there are herbs in the other honey recipes. It isn't because it makes it taste better, that is for sure! This is a medicinal honey that is popular during allergy season. We use turmeric honey by the teaspoonful for allergy symptoms and to get rid of a runny nose. Turmeric honey can also be put on the skin for sprains, strains, and bruises.*

1 cup (370 ml) honey

¾ cup (72 g) powdered turmeric

## WINTER COLDS HONEY

*Many spaghetti and red sauces for lasagna, manicotti, and other Italian pasta dishes call for sugar in their recipes. Instead of sugar, you can add 1 to 2 tablespoons (23 to 45 ml) of this honey to your red pasta sauce. Use it in your sauces, marinades, soups, and salad dressings to help keep away winter colds.*

1 cup (370 ml) honey

2 tablespoons (12 g) powdered garlic

2 tablespoons (12 g) powdered rosemary

1 tablespoon (4 g) powdered thyme

1 teaspoon (1 g) powdered sage

1 teaspoon (2 g) powdered oregano

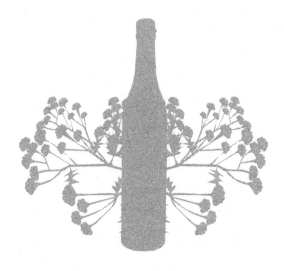

CHAPTER 7

# Herbal Vinegar

I love the diversity of herbal vinegars. Whether you use them to spice up your marinades or to soften your skin, herb-infused vinegars are great to have around. I guarantee that the few minutes that it takes to put them together will be well worth your effort. Most herbal vinegars have multiple uses. Basil vinegar is indispensable in salad dressings and a wonderful mood-enhancing additive in the bathtub. Juniper berry vinegar is perfect for wild meat marinades, or you can use it as a hair rinse to stimulate scalp circulation. Drizzle rose petal vinegar on fruit salad, or spray it on sunburns and acne. The kitchen and cosmetic uses of vinegar are limitless. I keep herbal vinegars in the pantry and the medicine chest, and we always have a large jar of some sort of herbal vinegar next to the bathtub.

Found in almost every home, vinegar can be used for much more than flavoring and tenderizing meat and vegetables. It enhances the nutritional value of any meal, heals the skin, and inhibits the growth of bacteria in food.

Vinegar is a superb medium for extracting minerals from herbs, fruits, and foods. Adding vinegar to bone marrow broths coaxes the minerals from the bones into the soup. Steeping herbs in vinegar pulls vitamins and minerals from the herbs, preserving them for meals in the coming season.

Herbal vinegars are easy to make and can add a variety of flavors to your meals that will continue to surprise and amaze those who eat your food. "What is in this sauce?" That may be a little difficult to answer. Not only does your sauce contain herbs and fruit that are specific to a particular season, but if you harvested the herbs yourself, sunshine, joy, fresh air, the conversation, and the beauty of the experience are also corked into that bottle.

Hand-harvested and home-crafted foods carry a memory and a feeling with them that is part of what makes them so special. How you feel and what you think about go into the food that is prepared. When I pour homemade vinegars into sauces and soups, I find myself smiling from the memory of creating them; that really does make your food more delicious. I enjoy being able to capture the fulfillment of summer's labor in the pantry and watch it unfold throughout the year in our lunch boxes and home cosmetics. When you have a bottle of vinegar that is infused with lemon verbena, lemon peels, blueberries, sage, and a bright summer day, inspired marinades aren't that far out of reach.

## GETTING STARTED

### SUPPLIES

Nonreactive containers with lids, such as sterilized glass jars

> Use a nonreactive container in which to make and store the vinegar. Glass, porcelain, or enamel work well. The lid of the container has to be nonreactive as well, so use plastic, cork, or plastic-coated metal or enamel lids. If the vinegar touches metal, it eats through it, and metal pieces drop into the vinegar. Plastic lids for Mason jars can also be found at specialty shops. You will also need a second sterilized jar when straining out the ingredients from your vinegars.

Wax/greaseproof paper

If you use a Mason jar with a metal lid, you will need to put two sheets of wax/greaseproof paper over the mouth of the jar before you screw the lid on.

Funnel

You'll need a funnel for the decanting process.

Muslin

Purchase white muslin from the fabric store that is thin but has a tight weave.

## INGREDIENTS

Vinegar

You can make herbal vinegars with any type of organic, uncooked vinegar, such as apple cider, white wine, red wine, or rice vinegar. I primarily use apple cider vinegar because of its many healing benefits, including its alkalinizing effect on the body and its skin-healing applications. Organic and raw apple cider vinegar is easy to find and is usually less expensive than specialty vinegars. There are several brands of apple cider–flavored vinegar, which consists of white vinegar with caramel coloring. Many stores carry this imitation apple cider vinegar product, so read the label to ensure you have real apple cider vinegar that is raw and unpasteurized. If you live near a wine region, you can find locally made vinegars that articulate an assortment of flavors to inspire your culinary vinegar adventures. Purchase vinegar that has not been heated during production. Vinegar that has not been heated or processed contains healing enzymes and is a much better product than more processed vinegars.

Herbs and Fruit

You can make medicinal and culinary herbal vinegars with fresh or dried herbs, spices, fruit, and berries in any combination. Normally I mix either fresh or dried ingredients together. There isn't a rule saying you can't mix fresh and dried ingredients together if you are motivated in that direction. I usually keep them separate because fresh-ingredient vinegars have a shorter shelf life than vinegars made with dried herbs and spices.

Honey

> I add honey to taste to decanted herbal vinegars (vinegars with the herbs strained out) that are going to be used for salad dressings. If you want to sweeten the vinegar, the following recipes require the herbs to be strained out first before adding a sweetener, unless otherwise indicated.

# MAKING HERBAL VINEGAR

## PROPORTIONS

The proportions used for making herbal vinegars vary depending on whether you use fresh or dried ingredients. The dried herbs and fruit have a stronger flavor than the fresh herbs and fruit.

¾ jar finely chopped fresh fruit or herbs

¼ jar crushed dried herbs or spices or finely chopped dried fruit

## METHOD

1. Prepare the ingredients: chop fresh herbs as finely as possible, crush dried herbs or whole dried spices in a mortar and pestle, or finely chop dried fruit.

2. Fill a glass jar with fresh or dried fruit, herbs, or spices according to the proportions listed above.

3. Pour vinegar over the ingredients, filling the jar to the top with vinegar. Make sure that the vinegar covers the ingredients by at least a couple of inches

4. If you are using a metal lid, cover the opening of the jar with two sheets of wax/greaseproof paper, and then put the lid on, or use plastic lids.

5. Store vinegar in a cool, dark place for one month. Shake it once in a while and occasionally check to see if you need to add more vinegar, as some of it may have been soaked up by the plant material. This tends to be more of a problem with fresh herbs and fruits than with dried. If the fruit or herbs are sticking out above the vinegar, add more vinegar.

## DECANTING

Depending on the ingredients in your vinegar, you may need to decant (strain out the herbs) after one month. If your vinegar contains only dried herbs and spices, they can be left in the jar for the duration of the vinegar use. Fruit and fresh ingredients need to be strained out after one month. Vinegars made for cosmetic uses can be concocted with fresh or dried herbs, but be sure to strain the herbs out of any vinegar that will be used topically.

1. Place a funnel into the opening of a clean, sterilized jar and lay muslin over the top of the funnel.
2. Pour the infusing vinegar through the muslin, being careful not to let the contents fall out of the side of the cloth.
3. Let all the vinegar strain through the cloth and funnel into the clean jar.
4. If your vinegar is made with fresh ingredients, don't squeeze what is in the muslin, or water will squeeze out of the fresh ingredients, giving you cloudy vinegar with a shorter shelf life. Just let liquid drip through.
5. Discard the strained ingredients into the compost. The liquid left behind is your herbal vinegar.

## STORAGE

Store herbal vinegar in a clean container in a dark cabinet out of heat, light, and temperature variation. Your vinegar should last for about one year. Make sure you store the vinegar in a container with a plastic or cork lid. The vinegar will eat any metal it comes into contact with. If your vinegar turns black, has floating chunks, or develops mold or a funny smell, throw it away.

# RECIPES

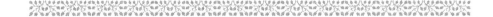

Herbal vinegars are a kitchen craft that vary greatly in the variety and amount of ingredients used. These recipes are general guidelines, but let your garden and the local harvest have its way with your creations. Dried spices such as ginger have a much stronger flavor than fresh herbs. I generally use more fresh ingredients per 1 cup (250 ml) of vinegar than dried ingredients. The following proportions are a general guideline. When using fresh ingredients, it is important to make sure that the vinegar covers the herbs completely.

## ACNE WASH

*This is a good home remedy for acne. Simply dab the vinegar on troubled skin twice a day. The vinegar smells and stings a little for a few seconds, and then it soothes and cools inflamed skin.*

¼ cup (24 g) crumbled dried rose petals
¼ cup (4 g) crushed dried lavender
¼ cup (4 g) crushed dried chamomile
¼ cup (48 g) crushed dried lemon balm
¼ cup (12 g) crushed dried rosemary
3 cups (750 ml) apple cider vinegar

## BLUEBERRY VINAIGRETTE

*Another creation that emerged from the garden. Everyone loved it so much that I had to remember how I made it; now it is a staple condiment in the kitchen. Mix this vinegar with olive oil to make a very satisfying salad dressing.*

1 cup (125 g) fresh whole blueberries
½ cup (24 g) finely chopped fresh lemon verbena
½ cup (48 g) grated fresh lemon peel

1 tablespoon (3 g) finely chopped fresh sage

1 tablespoon (2 g) finely chopped fresh parsley

3 cups (750 ml) apple cider vinegar

1 cup (370 ml) honey

> Let fruit and herbs infuse in the vinegar for one month, then decant. After the fruit and herbs are strained out, add the honey.

## BODY AND BATH VINEGAR

*Add 1 cup (250 ml) of this healing vinegar to your bath. It will rejuvenate your skin while helping you to relax.*

1 cup (96 g) chopped fresh lavender

1 cup (48 g) chopped fresh lemon balm

1 cup (48 g) chopped fresh rose petals

½ cup (48 g) chopped fresh rose geranium

¼ cup (30 g) chopped fresh burdock

5 cups (1¼ L) apple cider vinegar

## BRAISING VINEGAR

*After this vinegar steeps, it will thicken, and then you can spread it onto whatever you want to marinade.*

¼ cup (24 g) powdered orange peel

¼ cup (24 g) powdered coriander

1 tablespoon (6 g) powdered lavender

1 tablespoon (6 g) powdered black pepper

½ teaspoon (1 g) powdered horseradish

3 cups (750 ml) apple cider vinegar

½ cup (185 ml) honey

> Let the herbs steep in the vinegar for two weeks before adding honey. There is no need to strain the herbs from the vinegar, pour them along with the vinegar into whatever you are marinating.

## DRIZZLE VINEGAR

*This vinegar makes a great bread-dipping vinegar. Mix it with olive oil and fresh garlic and serve with warm sourdough bread as an appetizer.*

¼ cup (12 g) finely chopped fresh thyme

¼ cup (12 g) finely chopped fresh chives

1 tablespoon (9 g) minced fresh ginger

1 tablespoon (3 g) finely chopped fresh rosemary

2 cups (500 ml) white wine vinegar

## FIG DELIGHT

*Drizzle this vinegar on melons, fresh fruit salad, or sautéed summer squash.*

1 cup (185 g) finely chopped dried figs

1 teaspoon (3 g) minced fresh ginger

2 whole cloves

1 cup (250 ml) balsamic vinegar

¼ cup (93 ml) honey

> Let figs, ginger, and cloves steep in the vinegar for one month, then decant. After you have strained out the herbs and fruit, add the honey.

## FIRE CIDER

*This is an old favorite remedy for helping to sweat out a cold. Take 1 tablespoon (23 ml) of this cider three times a day at the onset of a cold.*

3 tablespoons (28 g) fresh grated ginger

2 tablespoons (19 g) fresh grated horseradish

1 yellow onion, finely chopped

4 garlic cloves, finely chopped

⅛ teaspoon (¼ g) powdered cayenne

4 cups (1 L) apple cider vinegar

Honey to sweeten

> Let ginger, horseradish, onion, garlic, and cayenne steep in the vinegar for one month, then decant. Add one-half part honey to sweeten.

## FIVE-FLOWER HERBAL VINEGAR

*Use any combination of lavender flowers, calendula petals, rosemary flowers, thyme flowers, sage blossoms, or rose petals. When people ask you, "What is in this salad?" and you say, "Five-Flower Herbal Vinegar," the only thing they can really say is, "What? What is that?" Then you use the opportunity to evangelize about the virtues of cooking with herbs. I feel like I have a treasure chest in my kitchen when the pantry is full of such enticing herbal condiments.*

3 cups (216 g) fresh, whole, edible garden flowers (see headnote)

4 cups (1 L) apple cider vinegar

## FOUR THIEVES VINEGAR

*Every herbalist has their own recipe for Four Thieves Vinegar. The story has it that grave robbers avoided the plague by using herbal preparations that included these herbs. This is one of the first herbal vinegars that I experimented with for medicinal uses, and we have been making it in my herb classes for years. The testimonials about ailments this vinegar has averted could fill a book.*

½ cup (48 g) finely chopped fresh lavender

½ cup (24 g) finely chopped fresh rosemary

¼ cup (12 g) finely chopped fresh sage

¼ cup (12 g) finely chopped fresh thyme

2 tablespoons (6 g) finely chopped fresh peppermint

3 garlic cloves, finely chopped

1 tablespoon (6 g) powdered black pepper

3 cups (750 ml) apple cider vinegar

## FRUITED VINEGAR

*Having a variety of fruited vinegars on hand is one of the tricks of making interesting and yummy salad dressings.*

¼ cup (47 g) finely chopped dried apricots

¼ cup (47 g) finely chopped dried cherries

2 tablespoons (4 g) crumbled dried lemon verbena

Dash of allspice

2 cups (500 ml) white wine vinegar

2 tablespoons (45 ml) honey

> Let the fruit, lemon verbena, and allspice infuse with the vinegar for one month.
> Decant the fruit and herbs from the vinegar before you add the honey.

## GARDEN VINEGAR

*Try this vinegar in potato salad, mashed potatoes, and creamed cauliflower.*

¼ cup (10 g) finely chopped fresh basil

2 tablespoons (6 g) finely chopped fresh rosemary

2 tablespoons (4 g) finely chopped fresh parsley

1 tablespoon (3 g) finely chopped fresh chives

1 teaspoon (3 g) grated fresh horseradish

1 cup (250 ml) apple cider vinegar

## GARDEN DELIGHT VINEGAR

*Sometimes I make vinegar with one fruit and one herb. Often one fruit along with several herbs find their way into vinegar, and then sometimes it is like making a soup—just throw in whatever is around and see what happens. Lavender, rosemary, rose geranium, rose petals, lemon balm, lemon verbena, peppermint, basil, parsley, thyme, and sage are all herbs that could be used in this recipe. As for fruits, I use those that grow where I live, like blueberries, strawberries, raspberries, blackberries, kiwis, plums, apricots, peaches, pears, pomegranates, persimmons, figs, tangerines, and oranges. Just about any fruit you can think of is a possibility. What grows near you? The fun is in experimenting with the bounty of contributions each season has to offer. This is a staple vinegar for salad dressings. You can't buy vinegar like this in the store!*

1 cup (185 g) finely chopped fresh fruit

½ cup (24 to 48 g) finely chopped fresh herbs

2 cups (500 ml) apple cider vinegar

2 tablespoons (45 ml) honey

> Let the fruit and herbs infuse with the vinegar forone month. Decant, then add
> the honey.

## HEADACHE VINEGAR

*Soak this vinegar in a washcloth and apply to the head and feet to calm headaches.*

¾ cup (72 g) chopped fresh lavender or ¼ cup (4 g) crushed dried lavender

¾ cup (36 g) chopped fresh peppermint or ¼ cup (24 g) crushed dried peppermint

¾ cup (30 g) chopped fresh basil or ¼ cup (24 g) crushed dried basil

3 cups (750 ml) apple cider vinegar

## HEALING BATH VINEGAR

*Add 1 cup (250 ml) of this vinegar to your bath to soothe the skin and promote healing and rejuvenation.*

3 cups (144 g) chopped fresh rosemary

3 cups (288 g) chopped fresh lavender

3 cups (144 g) chopped fresh lemon balm

4 quarts (4 L) apple cider vinegar

## HERBAL FACIAL TONER

*This herbal vinegar helps to tighten and tone the facial tissue without drying it out. Splash a little on after washing your face and then rinse it off. This vinegar can be used for inflammatory skin conditions such as acne and blemishes, and it can also be used for normal skin to give it a healthy and glowing appearance.*

¾ cup (72 g) chopped fresh chamomile or ¼ cup (4 g) crushed dried chamomile

¾ cup (72 g) chopped fresh elder flower or ¼ cup (4 g) crushed dried elder flower

¾ cup (36 g) chopped fresh rose petals or ¼ cup (6 g) crushed dried rose petals

¼ cup (24 g) chopped fresh calendula or 2 tablespoons (2 g) crushed dried calendula

3 tablespoons (9 g) chopped fresh sage or 1 tablespoon (6 g) crushed dried sage

4 cups (1 L) apple cider vinegar

2 cups (500 ml) rose water

>  Let herbs steep in the vinegar for one month, then strain them out and add to your compost or garden soil. Add the rose water to the vinegar.

## HERBAL VINEGAR MARINADE

*Adding herbal marinades not only enriches the flavor of your food, but the antimicrobial properties help to keep away colds and flu. I use more herbal vinegar marinade in the winter months, making our meals part of our preventive–health care practice.*

½ cup (15 g) finely chopped fresh parsley

¼ cup (10 g) finely chopped fresh basil

¼ cup (24 g) finely chopped fresh thyme

¼ cup (12 g) finely chopped fresh sage

1 tablespoon (3 g) finely chopped fresh peppermint

3 fresh bay leaves, finely chopped

2 cups (500 ml) apple cider vinegar

## JUNIPER REJUVENATION

*Put 1 or 2 cups (250 to 500 ml) of this vinegar into your bath to increase circulation and soothe sore muscles.*

½ cup (120 g) crushed dried juniper berries

½ cup (26 g) crushed dried rosemary

1 teaspoon (2 g) powdered ginger

3 fresh or dried whole bay leaves

2 cups (500 ml) apple cider vinegar

## LAVENDER–ROSE GERANIUM VINEGAR

*For a delicious salad dressing, add 2 tablespoons (30 ml) of this vinegar to ¼ cup (60 ml) olive oil.*

¼ cup (24 g) finely chopped fresh rose geranium

1 tablespoon (5 g) finely chopped fresh lavender

½ cup (93 g) whole dried currants

1 cup (250 ml) apple cider vinegar

¼ cup (93 ml) honey

> Add herbs and fruit to vinegar and infuse for one month. Strain herbs and fruit from the vinegar, add the ¼ cup (93 ml) of honey, and shake well.

## LAVENDER-ROSEMARY VINEGAR

*Put this herbal vinegar into the dinner marinade and then into your evening bath!*

¼ cup (4 g) dried lavender

2 tablespoons (7 g) dried rosemary

1 cup (250 ml) apple cider vinegar

Put herbs and vinegar in a clean glass jar. Cover the jar with wax/greaseproof paper and put the lid on. After a couple of days, check the jar to see if you need to top it off with more vinegar. Let mixture infuse in a cool, dark place for one month, and then strain out and discard the herbs.

## MINERAL TONIC VINEGAR

*Rich in minerals, this vinegar is the perfect condiment to sneak into soups, salad dressings, and summer smoothies. It is a mineral tonic vinegar and can be added to any meal calling for vinegar.*

¾ cup (42 g) chopped fresh dandelion leaf

¼ cup (38 g) chopped fresh dandelion root

      or 1 tablespoon (12 g) crushed dried dandelion root

¾ cup (23 g) chopped fresh parsley

¼ cup (60 g) chopped fresh oatstraw or 2 tablespoons (6 g) chopped dried oatstraw

3 tablespoons (18 g) chopped fresh chamomile

   or 1 tablespoon (1 g) crushed dried chamomile

1 tablespoon (3 g) chopped fresh peppermint

      or 1 tablespoon (6 g) crushed dried peppermint

¼ cup (30 g) chopped fresh burdock or 1 teaspoon (4 g) chopped dried burdock

¼ cup (47 g) whole raisins

4 cups (1 L) apple cider vinegar

## MUSCLE RUB VINEGAR

*This is such a good home remedy to have on hand, and it is so simple to make. It is very helpful to rub on after a workout or whenever your muscles feel tired and achy from overexertion.*

¾ cup (36 g) chopped fresh mugwort or ¼ cup (12 g) crushed dried mugwort

¾ cup (36 g) chopped fresh rosemary or ¼ cup (13 g) crushed dried rosemary

3 tablespoons (36 g) fresh juniper berries or 1 tablespoon (5 g) crushed dried
   juniper berries

2 cups (500 ml) apple cider vinegar

## PEPPERMINT RICE VINEGAR

*Use this calcium-rich vinegar to add a splash of yum to smoothies and iced tea.*

¾ cup (36 g) finely chopped fresh peppermint

1 cup (250 ml) rice wine vinegar

## RASPBERRY VINAIGRETTE

*Every time I make salad dressing with this vinegar, people ask me for the recipe. Mix 2
tablespoons (30 ml) of this vinegar with ¼ cup (60 ml) olive oil to make a crowd-pleasing
salad dressing.*

1 cup (125 g) whole fresh raspberries

½ cup (48 g) finely chopped fresh rose geranium

½ cup (24 g) finely chopped fresh rose petals

3 cups (750 ml) apple cider vinegar

Honey to taste

   Let the berries and herbs infuse with the vinegar for one month, then strain. Once
   decanted, add the honey.

## RED WINE MARINADE

3 cups (750 ml) red wine vinegar

¼ cup (12 g) chopped fresh rose petals

¼ cup (12 g) chopped fresh thyme

¼ cup (12 g) chopped fresh sage

1 tablespoon (6 g) powdered coriander

½ teaspoon (1 g) powdered cumin

½ teaspoon (1 g) celery seed

## ROSEMARY HAIR RINSE

*If you want your hair to be soft and really shiny, use this vinegar as a hair rinse after washing your hair. Simply pour a few cups of this rosemary vinegar into your hair, let it sit a few minutes, and then rinse.*

¾ cup (36 g) chopped fresh rosemary or ¼ cup (13 g) crushed dried rosemary

1 cup (250 ml) apple cider vinegar

## ROSE VINEGAR SUNBURN SPRAY

*This herbal vinegar is the perfect remedy for sunburns and itchy skin. Put it into a spray bottle and spray it on sunburns. The vinegar will sting the red skin for about a minute, and then it just pulls out the heat and soothes the skin. This vinegar also helps stop the itching from rashes and poison oak.*

½ cup (24 g) chopped fresh rose petals

¼ cup (24 g) chopped fresh elder flowers

1 cup (250 ml) apple cider vinegar

## SAGE VINEGAR

*Mixed with warm water, Sage Vinegar can cure a sore throat. You can also skip the honey, put it in a spray bottle, and apply as deodorant.*

¾ cup (36 g) chopped fresh sage or ¼ cup (24 g) crushed dried sage

1 cup (250 ml) apple cider vinegar

¼ cup (93 ml) Ginger Honey (page 165)

> Let the sage infuse with the vinegar for one month. Once the sage has been decanted, add the honey.

## TAMARI MARINADE

*For this recipe, you use organic tamari instead of vinegar. I fill several large jars and let it age for one year. The garlic gets soft and sweet, and you can eat it like candy. Use the sauce for rice and stir-fries.*

1 cup (250 ml) tamari

2 cups (180 g) whole peeled garlic cloves

1 teaspoon (3 g) minced fresh ginger

1 whole star anise pod

1½ cups (370 ml) Ginger Honey (page 165)

> Put all the ingredients into a jar at once, including the honey. Let age for at least three months before using.

## VINEGAR ALL-PURPOSE CLEANER

*Expensive green cleaning products seem to be the buzz; make your own and save some money!*

1 cup (250 ml) Lavender-Rosemary Vinegar (page 183)

1 cup (250 ml) hot water

¼ cup (87 g) vegetable-based liquid soap

1 tablespoon (27 g) borax

2 teaspoons baking soda/bicarbonate of soda

> Put all the ingredients into a spray bottle and shake until minerals dissolve. Shake before spraying and use to clean your house.

# CHAPTER 8

# Herbal Cordials

Learn how to make herbal cordials, and you will always have the most interesting parties. People stop asking you to bring food to the potluck and request that you bring the drinks instead! I make several cordials each season, so there is always one around for when we are invited to a gathering. I recently attended the fiftieth birthday party of a friend who is very involved in herbal education. Most of the people at the party use herbs in their everyday life; therefore many of them had special cordials tucked away for this type of celebration. No bar could compare with the drink menu that was offered that evening! There were dozens of sumptuous libations filled with seasonal fruits, spices, and herbal combinations that could only be created again in our imaginations.

Cordials are alcoholic herbal drinks that have a variety of uses. Cordials are often sipped before and after dinner as digestive tonics. There is always a cold and flu cordial around the house, and every year I make a big batch of sleeping cordial to help with those insomniac nights. Cordials are perfect for toasts at special occasions, to pair with foods and desserts, and to add that extra touch to seasonal feasts. I made several gallons of a very special cordial for my wedding. It was delicious and helped to create an ambiance that you can't purchase at the wedding-planning store.

It is so fun to get together with a friend and make cordials for holiday gifts and parties. You can find inexpensive, glass, or crystal cruets and canisters at dollar stores and thrift shops. Clean them well and then fill them with cordial for social festivities. People love it. I make holiday cordials and seasonal party cordials, and if there is a shower or special birthday party coming up, a custom-made cordial is in order for the celebration.

Cordials are high in alcoholic content and are meant to be sipped in small quantities. Cordial glasses are ½ to 1 ounce (15 to 30 ml) in size. If you start drinking a lot of cordial, the alcohol isn't that good for you, but a little sip before or after dinner can be very beneficial. Especially in the winter, there is almost always a little cordial on our table. I also love collecting cordial glasses and like to shop around at thrift stores for cordial glasses to give away.

Herbal cordials are also generous cooking companions. Add them to cakes and desserts just as you would vanilla extract/essence. Use them in marinades and glazes and put a dash into drinks. We add fruity cordials to homemade whipped cream and blend cordials into dessert fruit dishes. Cordial stirred into fresh fruit makes a tasty dessert that can be put together in just a few minutes. Cordials can be stirred into jams and other dessert sweeteners or sprinkled onto yams and vegetables before baking. Add some cordial to your next batch of chutney or pie filling, or put a tablespoon or two (15 to 30 ml) into morning pancake batter and French toast egg batter. During the cooking process, the alcohol precipitates off, leaving behind a melody of flavors for you to enjoy.

The first cordials I made were for sipping in the winter to prevent sickness. I left some of the cordials out in my cooking area, and they ended up in all kinds of things. I didn't go to culinary school; I just thought, hey, this orange ginger cordial would probably go well in a chicken marinade. Pretty soon, cordials were sneaking their way toward being a staple part of my cooking.

If you have a garden and fruit trees, your cordials are shaped by the land on which you live. When you have an abundance of something, it tends to become a fixture in your herbal concoctions. Every year is different in the garden; some years there are only a handful of apricots, and some years I have shelves full of apricot cordial, honey, and syrup. That is what I love about gardening; the pantry is inspired directly by the gifts of the earth.

# GETTING STARTED

## SUPPLIES

Clean glass Mason jars with lids

> When choosing your jar, use one that is the closest in size that will fit all of your ingredients with not a lot of leftover space in the jar.

Funnel

> A funnel is needed for the decanting process.

Muslin

> White muslin can be purchased at the fabric store. Use fabric that is thin and tightly woven. Thick fabrics soak up too much of your alcohol.

## INGREDIENTS

Drinking alcohol of choice

> You can make a cordial with just about any kind of alcohol. My favorite alcohols for making cordials are vodka, brandy, and port wine. I have friends that make cordials with rum, gin, and tequila. Never use rubbing alcohol; it is not for internal use. Often people ask me what kind of brandy or vodka I use. I buy whatever is on sale, and sometimes—especially for holiday and gift cordials—I buy the expensive stuff.

Fresh or dried herbs and spices

> You can make cordials with fresh or dried herbs. If you have fresh herbs, use them. If you can't get the herbs fresh, then it is fine to use dried herbs. Fresh and dried herbs can be mixed together.

Fresh or dried fruit

> Seasonal fresh fruit and dried fruits are also good cordial ingredients.

Sweetener

> Adding one-half part sweetener is what turns your tincture into a cordial. The sweetener can be plain honey, herbal honey, maple syrup, rice syrup, fruit concentrate, molasses/treacle, or stevia extract/essence. You can use a single sweetener or mix more than one together.

# MAKING HERBAL CORDIALS

## PROPORTIONS

The only difference between making a cordial with fresh versus dried ingredients is how much you put in the jar. Fresh plants contain water and take up more space, so you use more of them.

¾ jar finely chopped fresh herbs and fruit
¼–½ jar dried herbs and fruit

### MAKING A CULINARY TINCTURE

1. Prepare your ingredients: crush dried herbs in a mortar and pestle as much as possible. If using dried fruit, finely chop the fruit with a knife. Fresh herbs and fruit should be chopped fine.

2. Fill a clean glass jar with fresh or dried herbs and/or fruit according to the proportions above.

3. Pour the alcohol over the herbs and/or fruit, filling the jar to the top.

4. Put a lid on the jar, label the jar with the date and contents, store it in a dark place, and let the ingredients infuse for one month. Make sure your fruit and/ or herbs stay covered with alcohol. Occasionally check to see if you need to add more alcohol, as some of it may have been soaked up by the plant material. This tends to be more of a problem with fresh ingredients than with dried. Especially check your mixture the first few days after making it. That is when fresh herbs often absorb the alcohol, in which case you will need to add a little more alcohol to cover the herbs and/or fruit. The alcohol should cover the ingredients by at least 2 inches (5 cm).

### DECANTING

After the ingredients infuse for one month, you will participate in the ancient art of decanting (a fancy term for straining out the plant material from the alcohol).

1. Place a funnel into the mouth of a clean, sterilized jar and lay the muslin on top of the funnel.

2. Carefully pour the alcohol through the muslin and funnel, letting the muslin catch the herbs and fruit, and being careful not to let them spill into the jar. If the herbs and fruit spill into the jar, get a clean jar and start over.

THE HERBAL KITCHEN

3. Allow all the liquid to strain through the cloth into the jar. If you are using dried herbs or dried fruit, squeeze the rest of the liquid out of the dried plant material through the cloth into the jar. If you are using fresh fruit, do not squeeze the muslin, or you will end up with a cloudy extract. When making fresh fruit cordials, just let the liquid drip through the cloth.

4. Discard the herbs and/or fruit. Add it to your compost or just put it on the dirt in your garden. The liquid left behind is the herbal tincture and the beginning of your cordial.

## SWEETENING

Once you have decanted the herbs from the alcohol, you now have an herbal tincture that needs to be sweetened in order for it to be classified as a cordial. The amount of sweetener you put in is up to you. Traditionally, one-half part sweetener is added to one part tincture to make a cordial. Once you strain the herbs and/or fruit out, pour the liquid into a measuring cup to see how much you have. Divide that number in half, and that is the measurement for the sweetener.

## MAKING A CORDIAL WITH VINEGAR

Vinegar cordials are made in exactly the same was as alcohol cordials. The only difference is in whether you soak the herbs in vinegar or alcohol. I make vinegar cordials and use them in salad dressings and marinades. One thing to remember when making cordials with vinegar is that the cordial has to be stored in a jar with a cork or plastic lid. Vinegar eats metal and will corrode the metal lids.

## STORAGE

Because of their high alcohol content, cordials are viable for years. Cordials made with fresh fruit are the least stable, depending on the amount of water in the fruit. Plan on a shelf life of one year for fresh fruit cordials and a couple of years for everything else (but most likely they will disappear long before then!)

# RECIPES

The recipes below are guidelines; feel free to experiment with them, using what you have on hand and what is in season where you live. I make cordials with fresh and dried herbs and fresh and dried fruit. Fresh herbs contain water and take up more space in the jar. As indicated in the proportions guideline, fill your jar three-quarters with fresh herbs and fruits. The measurement for dried herbs varies greatly. Dried, pungent spices like ginger are much more potent than dried leafy green herbs, so use less of them.

Whatever recipe or proportions you end up using, always make sure that the alcohol covers the ingredients by at least 2 inches (5 cm). The fruit and herbs should not stick up above the alcohol. Remember to strain the herb and fruit ingredients out of the alcohol before adding the sweetener. The sweetener amounts are just a suggestion; adjust things to your taste.

Some of the recipes give exact proportions of ingredients; other recipes give you a list of ingredients with the parts indicated so you can make the amount that suits you. When the recipe lists parts, just chose how much one part is. One part can be 1 tablespoon or 1 cup. You get to decide how much cordial you think your family and friends will partake in! For example, let's say you choose a recipe, and you want your "part" to be 1 cup. One part would be 1 cup, and three parts would be 3 cups. These recipes are a place to jump in. Unleash your creativity and have fun experimenting with your own twist on the ingredients.

## AUTUMN'S BOUNTY

*This is a flavorful digestive cordial.*

1½ cups (188 g) whole fresh blackberries

1½ cups (278 g) finely chopped fresh pears

¼ cup (12 g) fresh finely chopped lemon balm

¼ teaspoon (1 g) cinnamon stick pieces

4 whole cloves

4 cups (1 L) brandy, or to cover by 2 inches (5 cm)

Pomegranate concentrate to sweeten

## CHRISTMAS CORDIAL

*This cordial makes a great Christmas present.*

2 cups (340 g) pomegranate arils

Finely chopped peel and fruit of 1 fresh orange

¼ cup (47 g) chopped pitted dates

½ teaspoon (2 g) powdered cinnamon

7 whole allspice berries

1 teaspoon (3 g) minced fresh ginger or ¼ teaspoon (½ g) dried ginger

¼ teaspoon (½ g) powdered nutmeg

3 cups (750 ml) brandy or to cover by 2 inches (5 cm)

1 cup (370 ml) honey to sweeten

## FRUITY FALL DIGESTIVE CORDIAL

*I love to pull out my collection of cordial glasses and have a sip of cordial for dessert.*

1 cup (185 g) finely chopped Granny Smith apples

2 tablespoons (12 g) finely chopped fresh orange peel

1 tablespoon (6 g) finely chopped fresh lemon peel

¼ cup (12 g) finely chopped fresh lemon verbena

1 tablespoon (12 g) whole raisins

1 teaspoon (2 g) chopped vanilla bean/pod

1 small cinnamon stick

3 whole allspice berries

2 cups (500 ml) vodka, or to cover by 2 inches (5 cm)

1 cup (370 ml) honey to sweeten

## HARVEST CORDIAL

*Homemade cordials make nice gifts. Package the garden's entertainment in a decorative cordial jar and have it on hand to give away.*

2½ cups (313 to 463 g) combination of fresh fruits such as peaches, nectarines, and
    raspberries, chopped

1 tablespoon (9 g) minced fresh ginger or 1 teaspoon (2 g) powdered ginger

¼ cup (24 g) finely chopped fresh rose hips or 2½ tablespoons (30 g) dried rose hips

¼ cup (12 g) finely chopped fresh rose petals or 2½ tablespoons (15 g) dried
    rose petals

4 cups (1 L) brandy, or to cover by 2 inches (5 cm)

Black cherry concentrate to sweeten

## SUMMER BERRY CORDIAL

*Blackberries and raspberries work well in this recipe, but use whatever berries you have access to. I have also used marionberries and currants. Add carbonated water and fresh lime juice just before serving.*

1 cup (125 g) whole fresh blackberries (see headnote)

1 cup (125 g) whole fresh raspberries (see headnote)

2 tablespoons (12 g) finely chopped fresh rose hips

3 cups (750 ml) brandy, or to cover by 2 inches (5 cm)

1½ cups (555 ml) honey to sweeten

## SUMMER SOLSTICE CORDIAL

*Port wine is already pretty sweet and doesn't really need extra sweetening. This cordial is a result of the summer's harvest where we live. See what grows near you and give it a try. Make a summer party cooler by putting this cordial over ice and adding seltzer water and fresh-squeezed lemon or lime juice.*

1 part finely chopped fresh or dried elder flowers

1 part finely chopped fresh or dried rose petals

1 part finely chopped fresh or dried lemon peel

1 part finely chopped fresh or dried peaches

¼ part whole fennel seeds

Port wine to cover by 2 inches (5 cm)

## SUMMER SPLASH PARTY CORDIAL

*Who needs to go to the movies when the garden is in full display? Relax and enjoy the garden's offerings.*

2 cups (250 g) finely chopped fresh strawberries

½ cup (40 g) fresh elder flowers or ⅓ cup (5 g) dried elder flowers

2 tablespoons (12 g) finely chopped fresh orange peel

2 tablespoons (12 g) finely chopped fresh lemon peel

1 tablespoon (3 g) finely chopped fresh peppermint

3 cups (750 ml) Chardonnay, or to cover by 2 inches (5 cm)

Honey to sweeten

Orange slice for garnish

> Let ingredients steep for a few days and then strain them out. Add honey and serve with an orange garnish.

## SUNSHINE CORDIAL

*With this cordial, I just walked through the summer garden and picked whatever herbs and fruit were ripe at the time. It turned out to be delicious. Use it for summer marinades and sauces. Drizzle on top of fresh berries or desserts or add a splash of it to an evening iced tea.*

1 cup (125 g) sliced fresh strawberries

½ cup (93 g) fresh nectarine slices

½ cup (93 g) fresh peach slices

¼ cup (24 g) finely chopped fresh lavender or 2½ tablespoons (2½ g) dried lavender

¼ cup (12 g) finely chopped fresh rose petals or 2½ tablespoons (15 g) dried
   rose petals

2 tablespoon finely chopped fresh peppermint

2 tablespoons finely chopped fresh rosemary

4 cups (1 L) rum, or to cover by 2 inches (5 cm)

Maple syrup and honey to sweeten


**RELAXATION CORDIALS**

## CHAMOMILE CORDIAL

*When my son was a toddler, he often had difficulty getting to sleep. I would give him twenty drops of this cordial in ¼ cup (60 ml) of water, and it would help him relax enough so he could finally fall asleep.*

½ cup (48 g) chopped fresh chamomile or ⅓ cup (5 g) dried chamomile

½ cup (56 g) fresh or whole dried fennel seeds

½ cup (15 g) fresh rose petals or 3 tablespoons (18 g) dried rose petals

2 cups (500 ml) brandy, or to cover by 2 inches (5 cm)

1 cup (370 ml) chamomile-lavender honey

## RELAXING LAVENDER CORDIAL

*This cordial can help you digest your dinner and relax at the same time.*

3 cups (216 g) fresh lavender

1 teaspoon (2 g) powdered nutmeg

4 cups (1 L) brandy, or to cover by 2 inches (5 cm)

2 cups (740 ml) honey, or one-half part, to sweeten

SLEEPING ELIXIR

*Everyone needs a little help getting to sleep now and then. If you don't need it, there is always someone you know who will!*

2 parts finely chopped fresh or dried chamomile

1 part finely chopped fresh or dried lavender

1 part finely chopped fresh or dried sage

1 part finely chopped fresh or dried lemon balm

Honey or molasses/treacle to sweeten

**DIGESTIVE CORDIALS**

 AFTER-DINNER MINT CORDIAL

*Have you ever wondered why restaurants serve after-dinner mints? It is ancient herbal wisdom at your service. Peppermint aids in digestion, and a little mint candy, if there is really some peppermint in it, can do the job.*

2 parts fresh or dried nectarine slices

1 part chopped fresh or dried lemon balm

1 part chopped fresh or dried peppermint

½ part chopped fresh or dried lavender

Cognac to cover by 2 inches (5 cm)

Maple syrup to sweeten

 ELIXIR OF HEALTH

½ cup (96 g) fresh hawthorn berries or ⅓ cup (25 g) dried hawthorn berries

¼ cup (24 g) finely chopped fresh orange peel
  or 2½ tablespoons (10 g) dried orange peel

¼ cup (24 g) finely chopped fresh calendula or 2½ tablespoons (3 g) dried calendula

2 tablespoons (14 g) whole fennel seeds

1 teaspoon (2 g) whole dried juniper berries

1 teaspoon (1 g) finely chopped fresh basil

½ teaspoon (3 g) grated fresh ginger

¼ teaspoon (½ g) powdered cardamom

2 cups (500 ml) brandy, or to cover by 2 inches (5 cm)

Orange peel honey to sweeten

## ROSE-CARDAMOM CORDIAL

*This dessert cordial is great added to ice cream.*

1 cup (48 g) finely chopped fresh rose petals or ⅔ cup (66 g) dried rose petals

1 tablespoon (6 g) finely chopped fresh lavender or 2 teaspoons (1 g) dried lavender

1 teaspoon (1 g) finely chopped fresh peppermint or ½ teaspoon (1 g) dried
peppermint

1 teaspoon (2 g) powdered cardamom

2 cups (500 ml) brandy, or to cover by 2 inches (5 cm)

½ cup (174 ml) maple syrup to sweeten

## THREE-SEED CORDIAL

3 tablespoons (21 g) whole fennel seeds

2 tablespoons (11 g) whole coriander

1 teaspoon (2 g) celery seed

1 cup (250 ml) brandy, or to cover by 2 inches (5 cm)

Fennel honey to sweeten

**COLD AND FLU CORDIALS**

We keep several cold and flu cordials on hand during the fall and winter. Anytime someone feels something coming on, they take a shot, and the cold never comes!

## ELDERBERRY COLD AND FLU CORDIAL

*I make several jars of this cordial every year, and we always run out. I give it away to students, family, and friends, and anytime someone feels a cold coming on, the elderberry cordial starts flowing. If you drink some at the very onset of cold symptoms, it can really keep the cold from progressing into a full-blown sickness.*

2 cups (290 g) fresh whole elderberries or 1⅓ cup (247 g) dried whole elderberries

2 tablespoons (19 g) minced fresh ginger

3 cups (750 ml) brandy, or to cover by 2 inches (5 cm)

Honey to sweeten

## NO MORE COLDS CORDIAL

1 cup (96 g) chopped fresh calendula or ⅔ cup (11 g) dried calendula

1 cup (145 g) whole fresh elderberries or ⅔ cup (120 g) dried whole elderberries

½ cup (48 g) chopped fresh rose hips or ⅓ cup (60 g) dried rose hips

2 tablespoons (12 g) finely chopped fresh orange peel or 4 teaspoons (5 g) dried
orange peel

1 tablespoon (5 g) whole dried juniper berry

1 tablespoon (9 g) minced fresh ginger or 1 teaspoon (2 g) powdered ginger

4 cups (1 L) brandy, or to cover by 2 inches (5 cm)

Black cherry concentrate and honey to sweeten

**SPECIALTY CORDIALS**

## APRICOT-CINNAMON CORDIAL

½ cup (93 g) diced dried apricots

½ cup (93 g) diced dried persimmons

½ teaspoon (2 g) cinnamon stick pieces

2 cups (750 ml) port wine, or to cover by 2 inches (5 cm)

## AVENA DREAMS

*This is one of the first cordials I fell in love with. Every spring the surrounding hills burst with
fresh oats. I pick them when the pods are milky and make this delicious nerve tonic cordial.*

2 ¼ cups (540 g) fresh oatstraw

3 cups (750 ml) brandy, or to cover by 2 inches (5 cm)

1 cup (370 ml) rose honey to sweeten

½ cup (125 ml) rose water to sweeten

Let oats steep in brandy for one month. Decant and add rose water and honey.

 ## CELEBRATION CORDIAL

1½ cups (188 g) whole fresh seasonal berries, such as raspberries and blackberries

¼ cup (24 g) chopped fresh rose geranium

¼ cup (10 g) fresh basil

¼ cup (47 g) pitted dried prunes

3 allspice berries

3 cups (750 ml) brandy, or to cover by 2 inches (5 cm)

Cinnamon honey to sweeten

 ## CORDIAL CAFÉ

*This makes a very tasty after-dinner cordial.*

½ cup (60 g) cocoa nibs

5 dates, chopped

2 tablespoons (12 g) finely chopped fresh orange peel or 4 teaspoons (5 g) dried
    orange peel

2 tablespoons (19 g) chopped almonds

1 vanilla bean/pod, chopped

Dash of powdered cinnamon

Dash of powdered cardamom

2 cups (500 ml) vodka, or to cover by 2 inches (5 cm)

1 cup (370 ml) allspice honey to sweeten

 ## CRAMP CORDIAL

*It is nice to have some herbal support for uncomfortable menstrual cramps. Try sipping
1 tablespoon (15 ml) of cramp cordial and then lie down and rest. For some people this
cordial can work wonders for troublesome periods. Part of the remedy is to rest. Don't drink
this cordial and try to keep going!*

1 cup (96 g) finely chopped fresh chamomile or ⅓ cup (5 g) dried chamomile

THE HERBAL KITCHEN

2 tablespoons (12 g) finely chopped fresh orange peel or 4 teaspoons (5 g) dried
   orange peel

1 tablespoon (12 g) cinnamon stick pieces

1 teaspoon (1 g) whole crushed clove

2 cups (500 ml) brandy, or to cover by 2 inches (5 cm)

Molasses/treacle and pomegranate concentrate to sweeten

## GARDEN WINE

*Possible herbs for this wine-based cordial include calendula, lavender, lemon balm, lemon verbena, mugwort, rose geranium, rosemary, roses, sage, and thyme.*

4 sprigs fresh aromatic herbs (see headnote)

1 bottle organic white wine

   Add the herbs to the wine. Reseal the bottle and let sit for several days before
   serving.

## LOVE POTION CORDIAL

*I enjoy creating distinctive cordials for special occasions. This illustrious cordial was concocted specifically for my wedding celebration. I put together the biggest batch of cordial I had ever made, and was it a sensation! Many years later I have people still asking me for this cordial. It is a good thing I remembered what I put in it. I hope you enjoy it.*

1 cup (48 g) finely chopped fresh rose petals or ⅔ cup (60 g) dried rose petals

½ vanilla bean/pod, chopped

1 teaspoon (4 g) cinnamon stick pieces

½ teaspoon (1 g) powdered cardamom

½ teaspoon (2 g) minced fresh ginger

2 cups (500 ml) brandy, or to cover by 2 inches (5 cm)

½ cup (185 g) rose honey to sweeten

¼ cup (87 ml) maple syrup to sweeten

¼ cup (60 ml) rose water to sweeten

## POULTRY MARINADE CORDIAL

*Make up a couple of bottles of this marinade to have on hand. It transforms your baked chicken into an epicurean feast.*

¼ cup (24 g) finely chopped fresh orange peel or 2½ tablespoons (10 g) dried orange peel

1 tablespoon (6 g) powdered mustard seed

1 teaspoon (2 g) celery seed

1 teaspoon (2 g) powdered black pepper

1 bottle white wine, or to cover by 2 inches (5 cm)

½ cup (185 ml) honey to sweeten

## RED MEAT MARINADE CORDIAL

¼ cup (60 g) dehydrated cane juice

3 garlic cloves

1 tablespoon (6 g) whole black peppercorns

2 teaspoons (8 g) whole mustard seed

1 teaspoon (2 g) fresh thyme

½ teaspoon (1 g) powdered cumin

1 bottle red wine, or to cover by 2 inches (5 cm)

## SPICY PEACH CORDIAL

*Add this cordial to whipped cream, or mix it into warmed butter and use it as a dessert topping. Splash it on stewed fruit or fresh fruit salad. Cook with baked yams, winter squash, and winter root vegetables such as beets/beetroot and parsnip.*

1 cup (185 g) sliced fresh peaches

¼ cup (24 g) finely chopped fresh rose geranium

1 tablespoon (6 g) vanilla bean/pod, chopped

3 cloves

Dash of powdered nutmeg

2 cups (500 ml) brandy, or to cover by 2 inches (5 cm)

Ginger honey (page 165) to sweeten

## VANILLA CORDIAL

*Make your own vanilla extract/essence and save yourself some money. Throw away the liquid imitation vanilla and enjoy your homemade liquid vanilla. This cordial can be used as cooking vanilla in cookies/biscuits and cakes, or add a splash to fresh cream for dessert toppings.*

2 vanilla beans/pods, finely chopped

1 cup (250 ml) vodka, or to cover by 2 inches (5 cm)

½ cup (185 ml) honey to sweeten

> Let the vanilla steep in the vodka for several months before using. You can leave the vanilla in the vodka for up to one year; just leave it in the jar while you use the extract/essence.

## VANILLA SPICE CORDIAL

*Use this the same way you would vanilla extract/essence in baking. I enjoy having some of the other flavors added to the vanilla. I use this in almond tortes, whipped cream, pies, and wheat-free baking.*

2 vanilla beans/pods, finely chopped

Dash of cinnamon stick pieces

Dash of grated nutmeg

1 cup (250 ml) vodka

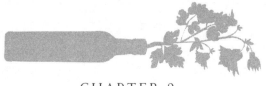

CHAPTER 9

# Herbal Oils

If you already cook with oils, why not add the extra therapeutic benefit of using oils infused with herbs? The nice thing about adding herbal oil to foods is that the flavor of the spice has been infused into the oil and is ready to liven up your meals. At least a half dozen herbal oils sit on my kitchen counter just waiting to be drizzled onto anything and everything. Infusing oils with herbs is such a simple way to enrich the taste and health quotient of your food. Thank you to the late Michael Moore of the Southwest School of Botanical Medicine for teaching me the fine art of making medicinal herbal oils. This single skill alone has shaped my life in more ways than I could have ever imagined.

The only two purchased oils in my cupboard are olive oil and coconut oil. Olive oil is on the table year-round, and coconut oil is preferred in the summer because of its cooling properties. We use oils made from locally grown olives that are organic and processed without heat or chemicals.

Many spices don't release their essence unless heated or blended into other mediums. Oil absorbs many of the flavors and medicinal qualities of herbs and spices. Having an array of infused herbal oils on your counter gives you a rich palette to draw from in creating your meals. When you add herbs and spices to food at the last minute, often there isn't enough time for the blending and synthesizing that can really elevate the taste. The aroma and flavor of herbal oil permeate food instantly. Just about any dish to which you add oil can be enhanced with infused herbal oil that pairs well with specific ingredients on the menu. Garnish your food with herbal oil; add it to salad dressings, sauces, soups, and stir-fries; and drizzle it over breads and marinades. It is useful outside of the kitchen as well, and is great for conditioning and moisturizing skin and hair.

# GETTING STARTED

## SUPPLIES

Clean, sterilized glass Mason jars with lids

Measuring cup

Muslin for straining

> Muslin can be purchased at the fabric store. Use thin, tightly woven cotton, as thick fabric will soak up too much oil.

Metal mesh strainer

Jar with sealing lid

Funnel

## INGREDIENTS

Organic Olive Oil

> Olive oil is a rich, nutritive, antioxidant, antibacterial, and cardiovascular tonic oil. It has a long shelf life, and I love using olive oil that is produced locally by people I know. It is not as stable as coconut oil when heated, but I still use it for quick sautéing. Olive oil is an indispensible ingredient in homemade skin and hair products. I have several herb-infused olive oils in my bathroom and use them daily in my self-care routine. Use olive oil that is cold-pressed and processed without heat and added solvents.

Organic Coconut Oil

> Coconut oil is pressed from the fruit of the coconut palm. It is solid at room temperature, liquefies above 76°F/24°C and remains liquid in warm weather. The changing seasons are always reflected in the jar of coconut oil. Coconut oil is an essential ingredient in healthful cooking and restorative skin care. It nourishes aged and damaged skin, conditions dry hair, and has anti-inflammatory effects when used topically and internally. Dr. Weston Price, the author of Nutrition and Physical Degeneration, found that the vibrantly healthy people of the South Pacific had traditional diets that were rich in coconut oil. Coconut oil is antibacterial, anti-inflammatory, and antioxidant. It is one of the best cooking oils, as it is more stable than most oils and doesn't oxidize at higher heat levels. Herb-infused coconut oils are more than delicious, they turn your food into a festival of vibrant, spirited nutrients with bold healing qualities. Purchase coconut oil

that is made from organically grown coconuts and processed without heat and chemicals.

### Dried herbs

Many of the spices can only be purchased dry; in that case, the oil is made with dried ingredients only. Dried herbs can remain in the oil for the duration of its use.

### Fresh herbs

Strain fresh herbs from oil after two weeks. When making infused herbal oil with fresh plants, mold can sometimes be a problem because fresh plants contain bacteria and water. If you harvest a fresh plant in the spring, when the water content is higher, it is better to let the herbs dry before using them. Don't harvest plants right after they have been watered or after a rain. If you wash fresh herbs before using them, be sure they are completely dry before making oil with them.

### 100 Proof Vodka

# MAKING HERBAL OILS

## PROPORTIONS

The following recipes can be made with fresh or dried herbs. Simply adjust the ratio of herbs to olive oil.

¼ cup (5 to 24 g) dried herbs per 1 cup (240 ml) oil
¾ cup (36 to 72 g) fresh herbs per 1 cup (240 ml) oil

### METHOD #1: DRIED HERBS WITH OLIVE OIL

4 cups (1 L) olive oil
1 cup (96 g) powdered herbs
1 to 2 teaspoons (5 to 10 ml) 100 proof vodka

THE HERBAL KITCHEN

1.  Powder dried herbs in the blender or purchase them powdered.

2.  Put herbs in a bowl and stir in the vodka. Mash and stir the alcohol into the herbs until all the clumps are worked out. Rehydrating the herbs with vodka enhances the extraction of medicinal properties and savory flavors.

3.  Put a sealing lid on the bowl and let rehydrating herbs sit for 30 minutes.

4.  Put the rehydrated herbs and olive oil in a blender. (Another option is to add the herbs and olive oil to a regular-size sterilized glass Mason jar and screw the blender base to the mouth of the jar. The jar can be inverted and used in lieu of the blender pitcher.)

5.  Blend herbs and oil together for 5 to 10 minutes, or for as long as the blender doesn't get too hot. If the blender starts to smell or smoke at any time, stop the blender and let it cool down completely. Once the blender is cool, blend oil and herbs together for 5 to 10 minutes until blender becomes warm.

6.  Pour oil mixture into a sterilized glass Mason jar (or if blended in jar, remove blender blade and screw on jar lid) and let sit for two weeks. Then your oil is ready to use.

7.  When making oil with dried herbs, it is not necessary to strain the herbs from the oil.

8.  Once you have used the oil, pour the remaining oily dried herbs into a marinade.

## METHOD #2: DRIED HERBS WITH COCONUT OIL

4 cups (1 L) coconut oil

1 cup (96 g) powdered herbs

1.  Powder dried herbs in the blender or purchase them powdered.

2.  Put oil and herbs into a sterilized glass jar and let it sit for 4 weeks.

3.  Occasionally shake the jar. If the weather is cold, coconut oil solidifies and needs to be stirred.

4.  When making oil with dried herbs, it is not necessary to strain the herbs from the oil.

5.  Once you have used the oil, pour the remaining oily dried herbs into a marinade.

## METHOD #3: FRESH HERBS WITH OLIVE OIL

1 cup (240 ml) olive oil

¾ cup (36 to 72 g) finely chopped fresh herbs

1. Chop fresh herbs as finely as possible.
2. Put herbs and oil into a sterilized glass jar.
3. Shake jar thoroughly several times during the steeping process.
4. Let steep for two weeks.
5. Decant herbs from oil (see Decanting Fresh Herb Oil, below).

### DECANTING FRESH HERB OIL

1. Place a funnel into the clean jar, then put the muslin on top of the funnel.
2. Pour the oil and infusing herbs through the muslin, being careful to not let the herbs spill over the side of the cloth into the funnel and jar. If the herbs spill out of the muslin into the jar, get a clean jar and start over.
3. When all of the oil has strained, do not squeeze the cloth, or you will squeeze water from the plants into the oil, compromising the shelf life of the oil.
4. Discard the herbs into the compost or put it in your garden dirt.
5. Shake oils before using.

### STORAGE

You can refrigerate your herbal oil to help preserve its shelf life. Remember that light, excess heat, exposure to moisture, and fluctuating temperatures break down the integrity of the oil. If the oil gets hot and cold, then hot and cold, the molecules break down more rapidly.

Infused herbal oils made from dried plants have a longer shelf life than oils made with fresh plants. Some herbs are highly antioxidant and help keep the oil from going rancid. Some fresh plant oils last for a week, and others are viable for months. Even the same plant can have a different shelf life depending on the time of year it is harvested. Develop your nose and learn what rancidity smells like. Smell all oils before you eat them or use them on your body. The following factors impact the longevity of your infused herbal oil:

the quality of the base oil

the amount of antioxidant properties in the herb used to make the oil

how your oils are stored

the quantity of water in the fresh plant

Dried plant oils are more stable than oils made with fresh plants. Herbal oils made with dried plants are good for one year. Herbal oils made with fresh plants have a variable shelf life depending on the antioxidant properties of the plant and how much water is in the plant at the time the oil is made.

# RECIPES

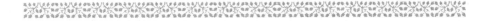

## AFTER-BATH OIL

*Oiling your body is one of the best things you can do for your nervous system. After-Bath Oil is rich in nerve tonic herbs that help to calm tension and anxiety.*

2 cups (480 ml) olive oil

½ cup (48 g) chopped fresh chamomile
or 2½ tablespoons (2½ g) crushed dried chamomile

½ cup (40 g) fresh elder flowers or 2½ tablespoons (2½ g) crushed dried elder flowers

½ cup (48 g) chopped fresh lavender or 2½ tablespoons (2½ g) crushed dried lavender

## ALCHEMY OIL

*This oil magically makes everything taste good! If I am in a hurry, I do a quick vegetable sauté with this oil, and the meal tastes as if I were in the kitchen for hours.*

1½ cups (360 ml) olive oil

1 tablespoon (6 g) powdered turmeric

1 tablespoon (6 g) powdered paprika

1 tablespoon (6 g) powdered coriander

2 teaspoons (4 g) powdered mustard seed

1 teaspoon (2 g) powdered cinnamon

¼ teaspoon (1 g) salt

1 teaspoon (5 ml) vodka

## CINNAMON-GINGER COCONUT OIL

*Enjoy the healthful benefits of coconut oil infused with this synergistic blend of healing herbs.*

1 cup (240 ml) coconut oil

2 tablespoons (2 g) powdered cinnamon

1 teaspoon (2 g) powdered ginger

1 teaspoon (2 g) powdered star anise

## ENERGIZER OIL

*Rub cold, tired feet with this stimulating oil, or use it to make a savory marinade.*

1 cup (240 ml) olive oil

1 teaspoon (5 ml) vodka

3 tablespoons (18 g) powdered chives

1 teaspoon (2 g) powdered mustard seed

1 teaspoon (2 g) powdered ginger

1 teaspoon (1 g) powdered bay leaf

## GOLD OIL

*I highly recommend this oil. Make up a batch and just see where it ends up in your dining experience.*

2 cups (480 ml) olive oil

3 tablespoons (18 g) powdered coriander

2 tablespoons (12 g) powdered turmeric

2 teaspoons (4 g) powdered fennel seeds

1 teaspoon (2 g) powdered fenugreek

1 teaspoon (2 g) powdered black pepper

1 teaspoon (2 g) powdered cumin

1 teaspoon (2 g) powdered mustard seed

½ teaspoon (3 g) salt

## INDULGENCE OIL

*This is one of my core oils that I use in everything from salad dressings and marinades to sautéing fish and vegetables. Try sautéing fish and vegetables in water and then topping it with Indulgence Oil just before serving.*

1½ cups (360 ml) olive oil

1 teaspoon (5 ml) vodka

1 teaspoon (2 g) powdered coriander

1 teaspoon (2 g) powdered fennel seeds

1 teaspoon (2 g) powdered turmeric

1 teaspoon (2 g) powdered lavender

½ teaspoon (1 g) powdered cardamom

½ teaspoon (1 g) powdered cinnamon

½ teaspoon (1 g) powdered ginger

½ teaspoon (½ g) powdered allspice

¼ teaspoon (1 g) salt

## LAVENDER OIL

*Mix a tablespoon (15 ml) of this oil into your salad dressing, or add ½ cup (120 ml) of this luscious oil into your foot soak. Massage it into achy muscles, or indulge in a lavender oil bath.*

2 cups (480 ml) olive oil

1½ cups (72 g) chopped fresh lavender

## LONG LIFE OIL

*This oil is so full of antioxidant properties and so delicious that even if it doesn't make you live longer, it will make you feel better. I sauté onions, garlic, celery, and bell pepper/capsicum in this oil as the starter for many dishes, including quinoa salad, jambalaya, garden medley stir-fries, and pasta sauces. It adds a note of full-bodied flavor when drizzled on steamed vegetables or fish.*

2 cups (480 ml) olive oil

2 tablespoons (12 g) powdered paprika

1 tablespoon (6 g) powdered coriander

½ teaspoon (1 g) powdered black pepper

¼ teaspoon (½ g) powdered star anise

¼ teaspoon (½ g) powdered nutmeg

## ORANGE JUBILEE OIL

*This is another marinade oil that has a central place on my lazy Susan. Right next to my stove, I usually have a half dozen herbal oils, a half dozen herbal vinegars, and several herbal ghees that just work their way into whatever is on the stove or in the salad bowl or blender.*

1 cup (240 ml) olive oil

1 tablespoon (6 g) powdered orange peel

2 teaspoons (4 g) powdered rose hips

1 teaspoon (2 g) powdered cinnamon

¼ teaspoon (½ g) powdered cardamom

## PAPRIKA OIL

*This is my favorite oil for corn on the cob. I once had a dinner guest just pick up her plate and drink the Paprika Oil that was left over from the corn.*

1 cup (240 ml) coconut oil

2 tablespoons (12 g) powdered paprika

¼ teaspoon (½ g) ground black pepper

⅛ teaspoon (½ g) salt

Dash of ground cayenne, or to taste

## ROSEMARY-THYME OIL

*This aromatic oil is great for marinade sauces. I use it as a cold and flu prevention oil in my cooking during the winter.*

1 cup (240 ml) olive oil

2 teaspoons (10 ml) vodka

2 tablespoons (12 g) powdered rosemary

2 tablespoons (8 g) powdered thyme

## SAGE-LAVENDER OIL

*This oil is good in marinades, pesto, and drizzled on bread.*

1 cup (240 ml) olive oil

½ cup (48 g) finely chopped fresh lavender

¼ cup (12 g) finely chopped fresh sage

## SAVORY OIL

*This is a delicious root veggie drizzle for baked parsnips, sun chokes, yams, and winter squash.*

1½ cups (360 ml) olive oil

2 teaspoons (10 ml) vodka

1 tablespoon (6 g) powdered rosemary

1 tablespoon (5 g) powdered parsley

1 teaspoon (6 g) powdered chives

1 teaspoon (1 g) powdered basil

1 tablespoon (2 g) powdered oregano

1 teaspoon (2 g) powdered lavender

¼ teaspoon (1 g) salt

## SEVEN HERBS MARINADE OIL

*This oil resulted from one of those experiments guided by the harvest of the day. It turned out to be a favorite marinade oil.*

4 cups (1 L) olive oil

⅓ cup (15 g) finely chopped fresh bay leaf

⅓ cup (10 g) finely chopped fresh rosemary

⅓ cup (15 g) finely chopped fresh thyme

⅓ cup (15 g) finely chopped fresh sage

⅓ cup (15 g) finely chopped fresh oregano

⅓ cup (30 g) finely chopped fresh lavender

⅓ cup (15 g) fresh peppermint

## SWEET AND SPICY OIL

*Use this oil to drizzle over baked fish.*

1 cup (240 ml) olive oil

1 teaspoon (5 ml) vodka

1 tablespoon (2 g) powdered allspice

1 teaspoon (2 g) powdered cinnamon

1 teaspoon (1 g) powdered thyme

1 teaspoon (2 g) powdered paprika

½ teaspoon (1 g) powdered black pepper

¼ teaspoon (½ g) powdered nutmeg

## SYNERGY OIL

1½ cups (360 ml) olive oil

3 tablespoons (18 g) powdered coriander

3 tablespoons (18 g) powdered paprika

2 teaspoons (4 g) powdered garlic

1 teaspoon (5 ml) vodka

## THREE TREASURES OIL

*Douse squash, potatoes, and eggs with this oil just before eating.*

1 cup (240 ml) olive oil

1 teaspoon (5 ml) vodka

2 tablespoons (12 g) powdered coriander

2 tablespoons (6 g) powdered fennel seed

1 teaspoon (2 g) powdered cumin

## VIBRANT LIFE OIL

*Put this oil on fresh corn instead of butter, or drizzle it on popcorn, steamed vegetables, or egg dishes.*

1 cup (240 ml) coconut oil

1 tablespoons (6 g) powdered paprika

2 teaspoons (4 g) powdered coriander

⅛ teaspoon (¼ g) powdered clove

# CHAPTER 10

# Herbal Ghee

Ghee is good for you! We substitute ghee in almost everything that butter would be used for. Ghee is butter that is heated in order to separate the water and milk solids from the butter fat. This process turns butter into a nutty, healthful, and nourishing food.

Ghee does not go rancid when you cook with it, so it is one of the best oils to use for baking, marinading, and sautéing. This liquid gold is also a great food for people who are lactose intolerant. Since the milk solids have been removed, ghee is suitable for those who need a lactose-free diet.

I love ghee, and as with every other medium in my kitchen, what do you think I do with it? Right! Add herbs. Ghee is a great delivery mechanism for the medicinal properties of herbs. Ghee carries the healing constituents of the plants deeper into the body, nourishing all tissues. It helps the body to absorb many healing qualities of the herbs while adding a wealth of variation and rich flavor to whatever you are eating. Add it to soups or the water you use for cooking rice and other grains. It is a delicious condiment on anything from fish and vegetables to popcorn and your morning toast. As my husband, Michael, says, "Anything tastes good with ghee on it." It also has cosmetic applications, and can be used as lip balm, massage oil for the feet and scalp, and a moisturizer for the entire body.

Start making your own herbal ghee blends, and soon the condiment aisle at the grocery store will pale in comparison to the creative flare of your home pantry.

# GETTING STARTED

## SUPPLIES

10–by-8-inch (25-by-20-cm) glass Pyrex pan

Stainless steel pot

3 sterilized Mason jars

Large glass measuring cup

Two 7-by-7-inch (18-by-18-cm) pieces of muslin

Large spoon

## INGREDIENTS

Unsalted organic butter

> Use organic unsalted, sweet butter. Use the freshest butter you can find and also look for pastured butter from cows that have eaten fresh green grass instead of grains.

Dried herbs

> Dried herbs for ghee need to be finely powdered.

Fresh herbs

> Fresh herbs for ghee should be finely minced. When adding fresh herbs to ghee, you put moisture back into it along with living plant substances. Now your ghee has a shorter shelf life than if it were plain or amended with dried herbs. Once I add fresh herbs to ghee, I like to use it within a week. Any ghee that contains fresh garlic needs to be used within a couple of days.
>
> Another handy way to use fresh herbed ghee is to put it into ice cube trays and freeze it. Once they are frozen, pop out the ghee cubes, put them in a lidded jar, and store them in the freezer. Whenever you need to add some life to your soup or beans, pull out a chunk of ghee and pop it into your meal. Frozen herbed ghee lasts up to one year.

# MAKING GHEE

I make ghee while I am doing other things in the kitchen. You need to keep an eye on what is happening so you can assess when it is time to move to the next step. Butter varies in its constituents and moisture content, so the timing for each step below will fluctuate.

Most resources for making ghee give directions to use a saucepan. I tried this for years. I burnt many batches of ghee, and it drove my students nuts because there is about a 30-second window when the butter fat finally turns clear before the curdy sediments burn on the bottom. Baking the butter in the oven first clears out most of the white curds on the bottom of the pan that can cause your ghee to burn.

## METHOD

1. Place a rack in the bottom-center of the oven and preheat oven to 275°F/135°C.
2. Unwrap 3 pounds (1½ kg) of butter (12 sticks) and put it in a glass Pyrex baking pan. Put the pan in the oven.
3. First the butter will melt, which takes about 30 minutes. The timing on this step varies depending on if the butter came straight from the refrigerator or if it was at room temperature before you put it in the pan.
4. Once the butter melts, bits of white foam will begin to congeal on the top layer in the pan. You will notice three layers of things happening: white creamy milk solids on the bottom, the golden butter fat in the middle, and the whey protein and moisture on the top.
5. Let cook for about another 30 minutes, and the top layer of foam will crust together and completely cover the pan. You want as much of this to bubble up as possible, without letting it turn brown or burn. If at any time things start turning brown or burning, remove the pan from the oven.
6. Once the white foam encrusts the top layer of the entire pan, carefully reach a spoon into the oven to scoop off the white layer and discard.
7. Bake for another 15 to 20 minutes, until another layer of white foam forms on the pan. Carefully remove the pan from the oven.
8. Scoop the remaining layer of white foam from off the top of the golden liquid and discard.

THE HERBAL KITCHEN

9. Pour the pan contents into a large measuring cup or pitcher. Fit a funnel lined with muslin into a sterilized glass jar, then pour the liquid through the lined funnel into the jar.

10. Let the butter fat drip through the cloth, leaving behind undesirable solids in the muslin. Once all the liquid has dripped through the cloth (do not squeeze), pour the liquid into a saucepan.

11. Over medium-low heat, cook the liquid for 10 to 15 minutes.

12. The liquid will simmer and bubble. Scoop the froth off the top and side of the pot with a spoon.

13. Stir, scraping the bottom of the pan to prevent anything from sticking there. Anything that sticks will burn and give your ghee an undesirable burnt flavor.

14. After 10 to 15 minutes, the golden amber liquid will become clear and the frothing will mostly stop.

15. Pour the liquid into a clean, dry measuring cup and then strain once again through a muslin-lined funnel into an airtight container. Your ghee is ready!

## ADDING HERBS TO GHEE

### Dried Herbs

For the following recipes calling for dried herbs, simply stir the herbs thoroughly into the ghee. If possible, add herbs to ghee while it is still warm from the process of making it. If the ghee has already cooled down, reheat the ghee on low heat until melted, add the herbs, and stir well. Once the ghee has solidified, stir the herbs again until completely mixed. Let herbs sit in the ghee for two weeks before eating. Do not strain the herbs out; eat the herbs right along with the ghee. Proportions are generally ¼ cup (24 g) of powdered herbs to 1 cup (240 ml) of ghee. This ratio varies significantly due to the diverse qualities of the herbs.

### Fresh Herbs

Fresh herbs can be added to ghee when the ghee is warm or after it has cooled down. Mix the fresh herbs thoroughly into the ghee. Once you add fresh herbs to ghee, you have reintroduced water, and the ghee should be stored in the refrigerator and eaten within one week. The general proportion guideline is ¾ cup (36 to 72 g) fresh herbs to 1 cup (240 ml) ghee.

**STORAGE**

The process of making ghee removes the milk proteins and moisture, producing a very stable substance. It does not need to be refrigerated and is stable for at least one year as long it is stored in an airtight container and moisture isn't reintroduced by leaving the lid off or splashing food and liquids into it. If you add dried herbs to ghee, it does not have to be refrigerated and is as stable as plain ghee. If you add fresh herbs to ghee, keep it in an airtight container in the refrigerator and use within one week. When using ghee, make sure the utensils dipped into it are clean and dry.

# RECIPES

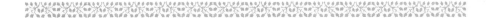

### GHEE WITH DRIED HERBS

## BAKING GHEE

*Add this ghee to your muffins, pancake mix, morning breads, and toast.*

1 cup (240 ml) ghee

2 tablespoons (14 g) powdered cinnamon

1 tablespoon (6 g) powdered fennel seed

½ teaspoon (1 g) powdered star anise

½ teaspoon (2 g) powdered nutmeg

## BLACK PEPPER–TURMERIC GHEE

*Add this ghee to your rice and grains, refry beans in it, and add it to any baked savory dish. This is a good winter cooking condiment, as the combination of herbs is antibacterial and helps dissolve pesky mucus.*

1 cup (240 ml) ghee

2 tablespoons (12 g) powdered turmeric

1 tablespoon (6 g) powdered black pepper

1 teaspoon (1 g) powdered bay leaf

## CORIANDER-CUMIN GHEE

*This ghee goes well with bean dishes, especially black and adzuki beans.*

1 cup (240 ml) ghee

3 tablespoons (18 g) powdered coriander

2 teaspoons (4 g) powdered cumin

## DIGESTION GHEE

*Fennel and black pepper are great carminative spices. Putting a dollop of this ghee on fish or rice dishes helps with digestion and adds an aromatic flavor that you will enjoy.*

1 cup (240 ml) ghee

2 tablespoons (12 g) powdered fennel seed

1 tablespoon (6 g) powdered coriander

1 tablespoon (6 g) powdered black pepper

## ITALIAN GHEE

*This ghee is a perfect base for red sauce. Sauté onions and garlic in this ghee as the foundation of spaghetti sauce. It adds a rich flavor to your cooking.*

1 cup (240 ml) ghee

2 tablespoons (10 g) powdered basil

1 tablespoon (6 g) powdered rosemary

1 tablespoon (6 g) powdered sage

1 teaspoon (2 g) powdered garlic

## LOVE YOUR HEART GHEE

*If you are new to making herbal ghee, make this one first. You may find yourself eating this ghee by the spoonful; it is almost as delicious as chocolate!*

1 cup (240 ml) ghee

2 tablespoons (12 g) powdered hawthorn berry

2 tablespoons (12 g) powdered rose hips

2 tablespoons (45 ml) rose petal honey

2 tablespoons (22 ml) molasses/treacle

## MORNING GHEE

*This is the best ghee for morning French toast, muffins, or quinoa. It is also a great addition to cornbread.*

1 cup (240 ml) ghee

3 tablespoons (21 g) powdered cinnamon

1 teaspoon (1 g) powdered allspice

½ teaspoon (1 g) powdered clove

## PAPRIKA GHEE

*Add this ghee to chili and stews, or put it in your slow cooker with your soup ingredients.*

1 cup (240 ml) ghee

3 tablespoons (18 g) powdered paprika

1 tablespoon (6 g) powdered garlic

## REJUVENATION GHEE

*Mix 1 tablespoon (15 ml) of this ghee into your rice water while cooking rice.*

1 cup (240 ml) ghee

2 tablespoons (12 g) powdered turmeric

1 teaspoon (2 g) powdered cinnamon

½ teaspoon (1 g) powdered ginger

½ teaspoon (1 g) powdered cardamom

## SAUTÉ GHEE

*Use this ghee for any soup or sauce that begins with sautéing garlic and onions. Sauté Ghee can turn any dish into a gourmet experience.*

1 cup (240 ml) ghee

2 tablespoons (12 g) powdered coriander

1 tablespoon (6 g) powdered paprika

1 teaspoon (2 g) powdered cumin

½ teaspoon (1 g) powdered clove

½ teaspoon (3 g) salt

 ## SAVORY SAUTÉ GHEE

1 cup (240 ml) ghee

2 tablespoons (12 g) powdered oregano

1 tablespoon (2 g) powdered sage

2 teaspoons (3 g) powdered thyme

½ teaspoon powdered cumin

½ teaspoon (1 g) powdered paprika

 ## SCARBOROUGH FAIR GHEE

*Add a teaspoon (5 ml) of this to soups, sautéed rice, and vegetable dishes, or mix it into cold grain salads such as tabbouleh, millet, or couscous.*

2 cups (480 ml) ghee

¼ cup (20 g) powdered parsley

1 tablespoon (2 g) powdered sage

1 tablespoon (6 g) powdered rosemary

1 tablespoon (4 g) powdered thyme

 ## SLEEPING GHEE

*Take 1 teaspoon (5 ml) of this ghee before bed for a peaceful night's sleep.*

1 cup (240 ml) ghee

¼ cup (93 ml) honey

2 tablespoons (12 g) powdered chamomile

1 tablespoon (6 g) powdered lavender

1 teaspoon (2 g) powdered fennel seed

¼ teaspoon (½ g) powdered nutmeg

## SOOTHING SKIN GHEE

*Apply this ghee directly to the skin. It helps to heal rashy, irritated skin.*

1 cup (240 ml) ghee

2 tablespoons (12 g) powdered calendula

2 tablespoons (12 g) powdered turmeric

## SWEET GHEE

*Infuse your foods with the cardiovascular-tonic and nerve-restorative benefits of roses.*

1 cup (240 ml) ghee

¼ cup (93 ml) Rose Delight Honey (page 168)

¼ cup (24 g) powdered rose hips

1 tablespoon (6 g) powdered orange peel

1 teaspoon (2 g) powdered cinnamon

**GHEE RECIPES WITH FRESH HERBS**

## BETTER THAN BUTTER

1 cup (240 ml) ghee

½ cup (20 g) minced fresh basil

3 cloves garlic, minced

## GREEN GODDESS GHEE

*This is a very scrumptious ghee for any savory food that you would top with butter or ghee.*
*It goes well with potatoes, baked bread, and any combination of vegetables.*

1 cup (240 ml) ghee

2 tablespoons (6 g) minced fresh chives

2 tablespoons (5 g) minced fresh basil

1 tablespoon (2 g) minced fresh parsley

1 tablespoon (3 g) minced fresh thyme

## PEPPER-CHIVE GHEE

*This ghee is delicious on warm sourdough bread. I like to dress up dinner plates with a decorative dollop of herbal ghee. Put some ghee into small candy molds, such as small flower- and heart-shaped molds, then pop them into the freezer for about one hour. Press the ghee from the molds and use it as the finishing touch on potatoes or vegetables.*

1 cup (240 ml) ghee

½ cup (24 g) finely chopped fresh chives

¼ cup (12 g) finely chopped fresh thyme

1 tablespoon (6 g) powdered black pepper

1 garlic clove, minced

## SAVORY GHEE

*Add this ghee to potatoes in all forms: mashed, baked, barbecued, or fried. Put it in potato salad or breakfast potatoes sautéed with onions and bell peppers/capsicums.*

1 cup (240 ml) ghee

¼ cup (10 g) minced fresh basil

2 tablespoons (6 g) minced fresh rosemary

2 tablespoons (6 g) minced fresh sage

3 garlic cloves, minced

CHAPTER 11

# Herbal Pesto

Creating your own herbal condiments is one of the best ways to indulge your creative cooking impulses. The combinations and variations are as diverse as life itself. Each season presents a smorgasbord of ingredients to heal your body and please your taste buds.

Pesto is more than a condiment in my kitchen; it is its own food group in our house. It holds a place as sacred as the elements—there is earth, water, fire, air . . . and pesto. It is so satisfying to make a batch each week and know that it is in the fridge to put on practically everything we eat. It is very rewarding to top off any meal with a creative, seasonal herbal pesto. And creative it is: using herbs is art in the kitchen. Turning your garden and spice cabinet into your food and medicine is an expressive art form and a lot of fun.

Pesto is a highly medicinal food, comprised of several servings of vegetables, loads of antioxidants, and a plethora of antimicrobial properties. People often limit their pesto indulgence to basil season. Well, there is more to pesto than basil. Don't get me wrong, I love basil pesto, but there are herbs you can use all year round to make pesto. For every season, there is an herb for your pesto. Throughout the year, we put pesto on eggs, toss it into bean salads, and mix it into pasta, soups, and stew. Add a little vinegar to your pesto and turn it into salad dressing. Spread it on pizza instead of tomato sauce, use it as a substitute for mayonnaise on sandwiches, or serve your guests raw veggies with pesto as the dip!

# GETTING STARTED

**SUPPLIES**

food processor

spatula

sterilized glass jar

**INGREDIENTS**

Olive oil

> You can use plain olive oil in your pesto, or experiment with infused herbal olive oils.

Garlic

> Pesto is a food, but having garlic as one of the main ingredients also gives it medicinal status. It is such a pleasure to have a medicine that tastes so good.

Fresh green leafy herbs

> The base herbs for pesto are arugula/rocket, basil, fresh cilantro, and parsley. I also use salad mix, lettuce greens, and fresh spinach as green leafy herb ingredients, but I don't use them alone; I always mix several of them together. The leafy green herbs are considered vegetable servings, so eat up. Don't you love the idea of getting some of your daily vegetable servings by eating pesto?

Fresh savory or stronger-tasting herbs

> Savory herbs such as chives, dandelion leaf, lavender, lemon balm, mustard greens, oregano, peppermint, rosemary, sage, and thyme add a heightened dimension of flavor to pestos, but if you don't fluff them out with the green leafy herbs, the pesto is too strong and can be overwhelmingly bitter.

Fresh edible flowers

> Calendula petals, cilantro flowers, fennel flowers, lavender flowers, rose geranium flowers, rose petals, sage flowers, and squash blossoms can all be added to pesto. Add ¼ cup (18 g) of edible flowers to a base pesto recipe.

### Dried spices

For the most part, pesto is made with fresh herbs, but it is also a great medium for sneaking dried herbs into your diet. Dried ginger, cayenne, paprika, cumin, seaweeds, and celery seed are a few of the dried spices that find their way into pesto creations.

### Cheese

Parmesan, Romano, and feta cheese go well in pesto.

### Nuts and seeds

Most pesto recipes call for pine nuts. You can also play around with cashews, macadamia nuts, pumpkin seeds, sunflower seeds, and walnuts.

### Salt

Any time you use salt, make sure it is the best salt you can get. We use pink Himalayan salt, gray Celtic salt, and a mineral-rich salt from Hawaii. Regular table salt is sodium chloride and simply not good for you.

### Spicy and sour ingredients

If you want to mix up the flavor of your pesto, you can add a small amount of one of the following ingredients to a batch of classic pesto: balsamic vinegar, capers, lemon, fresh ginger, Greek olives, fresh horseradish, jalapeño chile, or fresh lemon juice.

### Vegetable ingredients

Add variety to your pesto and experiment with avocado, baby kale, cucumber, chard, green/spring onions, red bell peppers/capsicums, or dried tomatoes.

# HOW TO MAKE HERBAL PESTO

**METHOD**

1.  Put the olive oil, garlic, and green leafy herbs into a food processor.
2.  Blend until you have a smooth paste.
3.  Add handfuls of other ingredients a little at a time until everything is completely blended.
4.  Put into a lidded jar and store in the refrigerator for up to one week.

**STORAGE**

Fresh pesto usually lasts in the fridge for about one week. We always eat it before then, but for longer storage, fill an ice tray with the pesto and freeze it. Remove the frozen pesto cubes from the ice tray and store them in a jar in the freezer. You can pull out a few pieces at a time to add to soups and sauces throughout the year.

# RECIPES

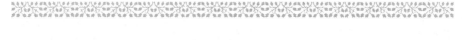

My basic pesto recipe does not include cheese. Once the cheese is added, it basically means that I can't eat as much of the pesto as I would like to. You will still find cheese in some of the pesto recipes, but they are richer and more suited for hors d'oeuvres and garnishes. I like to skip the cheese in main courses and eat lavish amounts of pesto.

Garlic varies greatly in gradients of heat, so you are going to have to be the judge of how much garlic you use. I follow the general guideline of adding one small clove for every 1 cup (30 g) of leafy green herbs.

# BASIC PESTO

¾ cup (180 ml) olive oil, or ½ cup (120 ml) olive oil

   plus ¼ cup (60 ml) herb-infused olive oil

2½ cups (75 g) fresh leafy green herbs

½ cup (24 to 48 g) fresh savory herbs

¼ to ½ cup (36 to 73 g) nuts or seeds

2 to 3 garlic cloves

¼ teaspoon (1 g) salt

## Variations

¼ cup (31 g) grated Parmesan or Romano cheese

## More variations

Add one of the following ingredients to the Basic Pesto recipe for variety.

¼ cup (18 g) fresh edible flowers (see Fresh Edible Flowers, page 227)

¼ cup (23 g) chopped dry-packed sun-dried tomato

1 green/spring onion (white and green parts)

1 red bell pepper/capsicum

¼ cup (39 g) whole Greek olives, pitted

¼ cup (75 g) capers

1 to 2 tablespoons (15 to 30 ml) fresh lemon juice

1 tablespoon (15 ml) balsamic vinegar

1 tablespoon (15 ml) tamari

1 teaspoon (3 g) fresh grated ginger

1 teaspoon (3 g) fresh grated horseradish

Cayenne to taste

Jalapeño chiles to taste

## ANTI-PLAGUE PESTO

*Embalm yourself with this pesto, and you won't have to worry about whatever flu is going around. I like this pesto on eggs and toast for breakfast.*

¾ cup (180 ml) olive oil

1 cup (30 g) fresh basil

1 cup (30 g) fresh parsley

¼ cup (12 g) fresh rosemary

¼ cup (12 g) fresh oregano

2 tablespoons (9 g) fresh lavender

3 garlic cloves

¼ cup (39 g) pine nuts

¼ cup (31 g) grated Parmesan cheese

1 green/spring onion (white and green parts)

½ teaspoon (3 g) salt

## ARUGULA–PUMPKIN SEED PESTO

*Pumpkin seeds are a healthy addition to the invigorating ingredients in pesto. Pumpkin seeds are a rich source of minerals including iron, magnesium, and zinc. They contain healthful omega-3 oils that feed the brain and promote overall wellness.*

¾ cup (180 ml) olive oil

2 cups (60 g) arugula/rocket

½ cup (15 g) fresh parsley

¼ cup (24 g) fresh thyme

½ cup (69 g) pumpkin seeds

½ cup (45 g) dry-packed chopped sun-dried tomatoes

3 garlic cloves

2 teaspoons (10 ml) balsamic vinegar

½ teaspoon (3 g) salt

## ARUGULA-SAGE PESTO

*Arugula and sage grow all winter long in my garden. Although I love basil pesto, I don't miss it in the winter because I also love this one.*

¾ cup (180 ml) olive oil

2½ cups (75 g) arugula/rocket

½ cup (15 g) fresh parsley

¼ cup (24 g) fresh sage

2 garlic cloves

¼ cup (31 g) sunflower seeds

¼ cup (31 g) grated Romano cheese

Dash of salt

Dash of powdered black pepper

## CILANTRO PESTO

*This is a more piquant-tasting pesto that provides an explosion of flavor to pasta dishes.*

½ cup (120 ml) olive oil

2½ cups (75 g) cilantro

1 cup (30 g) spinach

½ cup (24 g) chopped fresh chives

¼ cup (31 g) walnuts

1 garlic clove

4 teaspoons (20 ml) fresh lemon juice

¼ teaspoon (1 g) salt

## CLASSIC PESTO

¾ cup (180 ml) olive oil

3 cups (90 g) fresh basil

3 garlic cloves

¼ cup (39 g) pine nuts

½ cup (63 g) grated Parmesan cheese

Salt and pepper to taste

## FLOWER PESTO

*I love edible flowers. My son has obviously taken note. When we visit a place that has an unfamiliar flower, he asks, "Is this edible, Mommy?" Some flowers are poisonous, so it is good to be sure of which ones you can eat.*

½ cup (120 ml) olive oil

2 cups (60 g) fresh basil

½ cup (36 g) fresh edible flowers (see Fresh Edible Flowers, page 227)

¼ cup (8 g) fresh parsley

2 garlic cloves

¼ cup (42 g) cashews

1 tablespoon (19 g) capers

2 teaspoons (10 ml) tamari

## OREGANO PESTO

*Use this pesto to top off a fish dish, add it to tacos, or stir it into steamed veggies.*

¾ cup (180 ml) olive oil, or ½ cup (120 ml) olive oil plus ¼ cup (60 ml) oregano-
     infused olive oil

1 cup (30 g) arugula/rocket

1 cup (30 g) mixed/salad greens

½ cup (48 g) fresh oregano

½ cup (78 g) diced cucumber

½ cup (84 g) cashews

1 avocado

3 garlic cloves

1 tablespoon (15 ml) tamari

¼ teaspoon (1 g) salt

¼ teaspoon (½ g) powdered black pepper

## PESTO PICANTE

*Some people enjoy a spicy pesto; add more or less jalapeno and cayenne depending on your preference for spiciness.*

½ cup (120 ml) olive oil

¼ cup (60 ml) Rosemary-Thyme Oil (page 213)

2 cups (60 g) fresh basil

1 cup (30 g) arugula/rocket

¼ cup (12 g) fresh rosemary

½ cup (63 g) sunflower seeds

3 tomatillos

1 jalapeño chile, seeded

1 garlic clove

1 teaspoon (3 g) minced fresh ginger

½ teaspoon (1 g) powdered cayenne

Dash of salt

## PESTO REVIVAL

½ cup (120 ml) olive oil

1 cup (30 g) fresh basil leaves

1 cup (30 g) spinach

¼ cup (24 g) fresh thyme

¼ cup (12 g) chopped fresh chives

¼ cup (24 g) fresh lemon balm

2 garlic cloves

¼ cup (31 g) sunflower seeds

¼ cup (31 g) Parmesan cheese

1 tablespoon (15 ml) balsamic vinegar

Dash of salt

## ROSEMARY PESTO

*Think of your rosemary pesto as something that actually belongs in the medicine cabinet! It fights coughs, cold, flu, brain fog, forgetfulness, and fatigue.*

½ cup (120 ml) olive oil

1 cup (30 g) arugula/rocket

1 cup (30 g) mixed/salad greens

½ cup (24 g) fresh rosemary

½ cup (15 ml) fresh parsley

2 garlic cloves

¼ cup (42 g) cashews

½ cup (63 g) grated Parmesan cheese

½ teaspoon (1 g) powdered paprika

¼ teaspoon (1 g) sea salt

¼ teaspoon (½ g) ground black pepper

1 teaspoon (5 ml) balsamic vinegar

## SUMMER GARDEN PESTO

½ cup (120 ml) olive oil

1 cup (30 g) fresh basil

½ cup (28 g) fresh dandelion leaf

½ cup (15 g) fresh parsley

½ cup (24 g) chopped fresh chives

½ cup (36 to 48 g) of a combination of fresh sage, lavender, and thyme

1 green/spring onion (both white and green parts)

2 garlic cloves

1 red bell pepper

¼ cup (31 g) grated Parmesan cheese

¼ cup (31 g) sunflower seeds

2 teaspoons (10 ml) tamari

## ZESTY PESTO

*This is also called spring pesto; I make it with the first plants that come up in the spring. It is such a joy to gather the first green things of the season to make a fresh pesto. The basil is not ready yet, but there is usually still parsley left over from the winter, and the mustard greens growing everywhere in the hills let you know that it is time to make spring pesto.*

½ cup (120 ml) olive oil

2 cups (112 g) chopped mustard greens

1 cup (30 g) fresh parsley

½ cup (78 g) pine nuts

1 to 2 garlic cloves

¼ (1 g) teaspoon salt

¼ teaspoon (½ g) powdered black pepper

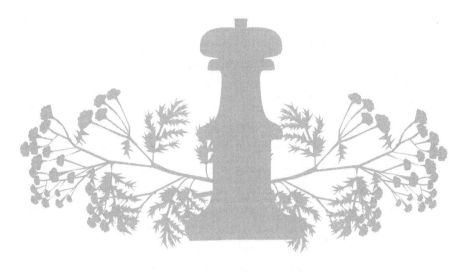

CHAPTER 12

# Herbal Sprinkles and Salts

This is one of the most simple and satisfying ways to incorporate more herbs into your cookery. The key to using herbal sprinkles is to have a dozen of them made up and located next to where you cook. Get twelve jars that are the same size and fit on a rack or shelf next to your stove. I like 4- or 8-ounce jars. If you are new to using lots of dried seasonings, begin with a dozen powdered herbs and use them individually. Get to know the herbs, find out what you like, how much you like, and what they taste good with. After a while, you just naturally want to mix more than one spice together.

I usually have three or four savory sprinkle blends for salad dressings, rubs, and marinades; several sweet and aromatic blends that are used lavishly in breakfast foods and treats; and then a few blends that contain specific healing herbs that I want more of in my diet. The specialty blends like Love Your Liver (page 245) or Turmeric-Ginger Sprinkle (page 247) can easily be added to drinks, smoothies, and breakfast foods. I just slip them in as many places as present themselves. You can add dried herb mixtures to recipes that call for flour, like pie crust, muffins, dumplings, and cornbread. Just add some of the herbs to the flour when making the batter. I also put powdered herb mixtures into whatever fruit and nut snack combination that is drying in the dehydrator.

I keep several sprinkles on lazy Susans next to my cooking area and on the kitchen table. If the herbs are readily accessible, you get into the habit of using them, and then pretty soon you wonder how you lived without such a pleasing array of sensory enhancement.

The title of this chapter could be "Beyond Salt and Pepper." No matter where you go, there are two herbs that decorate the table: salt and pepper. I find it fascinating that we settled on these two substances to adorn tables in eating establishments everywhere. I got the idea of having more options to choose from while dining with my Persian friends. They have salt and pepper, but they always have a third shaker that is filled with sumac. Pizza parlors also have dried chile in a shaker, but I take it a step further with at least seven shakers on my table at a given time! If the herbs are out and on the table, people are more likely to use them. Kids have fun searching the sprinkles for what goes best with their meal. I fill the shakers each season, adjusting the contents for the coming weather.

Some herb sprinkles are in regular salt and pepper shakers, and others are in shakers with larger holes, such as the shakers in which you commonly find chile flakes. I have a few other shakers with hole sizes that are somewhere in between the salt shaker and the chile flake shaker. We also have several tiny bowls with miniature serving spoons filled with herbs. Children love to use the small spoons. The best place to find various herb shakers are at professional kitchen supply or culinary specialty stores.

The kitchen herbs are abundant in their healing gifts and nutritional benefits. These herbal sprinkle mixtures bring the healing qualities of your spice cabinet to the center of your daily culinary experience. Enjoy this wonderfully creative and delicious journey.

# GETTING STARTED

**SUPPLIES**

Jar with tight-fitting lid for herbed salts

Salt shaker for herbal sprinkles

**INGREDIENTS**

Finely powdered herbs

> The herbs and spices used in shakers need to be finely powdered. Home powdering isn't sufficient for most spices. The blenders aren't powerful enough to completely break them down. There is the tendency to grind them for too long, and the heat generated by the blender dissipates beneficial components of the spices. Also, the small sticks and seeds get caught in the holes and clog up your shaker. Some dried herbs such as pepper and coriander can be left whole and put in a pepper grinder and used that way. Leafy green herbs such as basil, peppermint, parsley, and chives powder up well in a home blender. If you aren't growing your leafy spices, purchase them dried in whole form and then powder them in the blender.

High-quality mineral salt

> Use the highest-quality salt that you can find. Regular table salt is sodium chloride, which can trigger a litany of health problems. Whole salt is a healthful condiment that is teeming with minerals. Celtic salt, pink salt, gray salt, and Himalayan salt are some of the high-quality salts that are available.

# MAKING HERBAL SPRINKLES AND SALTS

**METHOD**

1.  Purchase powdered herbs and spices, or grind homegrown leafy green herbs in a blender. Sesame seeds can be used whole.

2.  Mix herbs together well in a bowl. Put the mixed herbs into a shaker or chosen dispenser for sprinkling on your food. Easy! If you want to use herb blends in a soup, put them in a bouquet garni pouch or wrap them in a piece of muslin tied with a string. You can keep this little bundle in the pot the entire time the soup is cooking. Herb sprinkles can also be turned into pastes by adding just enough olive oil to the sprinkle to make a paste. Herb pastes can be used for marinades and crusts for meats, vegetables, and fish.

**STORAGE**

The shakers have open holes, so the herbs are constantly exposed to oxygen. This exposure breaks down the herbs more rapidly, but they still last pretty well in the shaker, and usually six months isn't a problem. I prefer shakers with lids that close over the holes when you are finished using them.

If you keep your herb salts in a jar with a tight-fitting lid, they can last for one year and sometimes longer. What happens with salt is you start rubbing your food with it and leave it open while you are cooking. The salt and herbs cake together if they are exposed to moisture or if other foodstuffs get into the salt.

# RECIPES

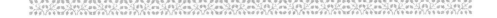

## HERBAL SPRINKLE RECIPES

Here are many of the herb combinations that are favorites at our table.

## AFTER-DINNER SEED CHEW

*We keep this seed chew on our kitchen table, and I also have a small container of it in the car. Food that we eat while traveling isn't as pure as what we eat at home, so we chew on these seeds to help us with a traveler's tummy. Many people experience constipation or a cranky belly when they eat away from home. This is the perfect remedy for the road.*

2 tablespoons (50 g) whole sesame seeds

2 tablespoons (14 g) whole fennel seeds

1 teaspoon (2 g) whole cumin seeds

## ANTIBACTERIAL SPRINKLE

*Consider it preventive medicine when you add antibacterial herbs to your spaghetti and meatballs. This antibacterial sprinkle goes into almost all our meat dishes. When we add antibacterial herbs to our food, we help our body not to have to do all the work!*

1 tablespoon (6 g) powdered rosemary

1 tablespoon (1 g) powdered thyme

1 teaspoon (2 g) powdered fennel seed

## BAKING HERBS

*Add this herb mixture to sweet breads, pie, cake, muffins, and other desserts.*

¼ cup (28 g) powdered cinnamon

2 tablespoons (12 g) powdered coriander

¾ teaspoon (1½ g) powdered cloves

½ teaspoon (1 g) powdered ginger

¼ teaspoon (½ g) powdered nutmeg

## BARBECUE SPRINKLE

*Dry-rub meats, potatoes, or vegetables with this sprinkle before grilling them on the barbecue. Dry-rub meat before baking, and then make gravy with the pan drippings.*

2 tablespoons (12 g) powdered coriander

1 tablespoon (6 g) powdered paprika

1 tablespoon (6 g) powdered black pepper

1 teaspoon (2 g) powdered cumin

½ teaspoon (1 g) powdered clove

## BREAKFAST SPRINKLE

*Toast, French toast, muffins, scones, bagels, and creamed rice all taste better with a dash of this sprinkle. If you feel like you are catching a cold, mix this sprinkle with enough olive oil to make a paste. Rub the paste into your feet and put socks on over the paste for twenty minutes. The antibacterial properties will flood your bloodstream and help you to fight off a cold.*

3 tablespoons (21 g) powdered cinnamon

1 tablespoon (2 g) powdered allspice

½ teaspoon (1 g) powdered clove

## CORIANDER SPRINKLE

*I sprinkle this on sautéed vegetables and rice, and it is especially tasty on eggplant/aubergine.*

2 tablespoons (12 g) powdered coriander

2 teaspoons (4 g) powdered cumin

¼ teaspoon (½ g) powdered cayenne

## CRUSTING BLEND

*Pack meat or vegetables with this blend and then bake it in the oven.*

1 cup (400 g) sesame seeds

½ cup (32 g) powdered thyme

½ cup (48 g) powdered rose hips

1 teaspoon (2 g) powdered black pepper

# DIGESTIVE SUPPORT SPRINKLE

*We always have Digestive Support Sprinkle to put on toast, hot cereals, or to mix into yogurt. The digestive support herbs are an incredible resource for daily health and well-being, as they help us to more efficiently digest the nutrients in our food. Whenever I add the Digestive Support Sprinkle to my cooking, I think of the prevention and healing it is providing my family. Your thoughts can potentiate the actions of herbs. The next time you add spices to your food, visualize your family in your mind's eye and imagine them healthy and happy.*

3 tablespoons (31 g) powdered flax seeds

2 tablespoons (14 g) powdered cinnamon

1 teaspoon (2 g) powdered ginger

½ teaspoon (1 g) powdered cardamom

# GARDEN MEAT RUB

*This rub helps to tenderize and flavor your meat before cooking.*

¼ cup (63 g) salt

3 tablespoons (18 g) powdered rosemary

3 tablespoons (18 g) powdered orange peel

2 tablespoons (8 g) powdered thyme

1 tablespoon (2 g) powdered sage

1 tablespoon (6 g) powdered black pepper

1 teaspoon (2 g) powdered horseradish

# GARDEN SALT SUBSTITUTE

*The Garden Salt Substitute is delicious on grains, potatoes, and rice dishes.*

3 tablespoons (18 g) powdered chives

2 tablespoons (10 g) powdered parsley

2 teaspoons (4 g) powdered rosemary

2 teaspoons (3 g) powdered thyme

½ teaspoon (1 g) celery seed

## HAPPY LIFE SEASONING

*Add this seasoning to marinades, salad dressings, and sautés. It is an all-purpose seasoning that has graced most every dinner that I cook. If I can't think of what to do with a dish, I add Happy Life Seasoning!*

1 tablespoon (6 g) powdered fennel seed

1 tablespoon (6 g) powdered lavender

1 tablespoon (6 g) powdered rose petals

½ teaspoon (1 g) powdered cinnamon

¼ teaspoon (½ g) powdered nutmeg

¼ teaspoon (½ g) powdered clove

¼ teaspoon (½ g) powdered ginger

## HERBAL MARINADE MIXTURE

1 tablespoon (5 g) powdered basil

1 teaspoon (2 g) powdered rosemary

1 teaspoon (1 g) powdered thyme

1 teaspoon (2 g) powdered garlic

1 teaspoon (2 g) powdered black pepper

1 teaspoon (2 g) powdered paprika

## HERBES DE CALIFORNIA

*Make up ten little pouches of this herb mixture. Wrap the herbs in small square pieces of muslin and tie them with string. Put into soups, stews, or foot baths.*

2 tablespoons (12 g) powdered lavender

2 tablespoons (12 g) powdered rosemary

1 tablespoon (6 g) powdered fennel seed

1 tablespoon (6 g) powdered calendula

½ teaspoon (6 g) powdered peppermint

## LOVE YOUR LIVER SPRINKLE

*Sprinkle this nourishing mixture into smoothies and salad dressings.*

2 tablespoons (50 g) sesame seeds

2 tablespoons (12 g) powdered dandelion leaf

1 teaspoon (2 g) powdered dandelion root

1 teaspoon (2 g) powdered burdock

1 teaspoon (1 g) powdered parsley

1 teaspoon (1 g) powdered seaweed (wakame, kombu, or dulse)

## ORANGE SPICE SPRINKLE

*This sprinkle is delicious in homemade applesauce, or add it to puréed fruits when making fruit leather in a dehydrator.*

2 tablespoons (12 g) powdered orange peel

1 tablespoon (6 g) powdered fennel seed

½ teaspoon (1 g) powdered ginger

¼ teaspoon (½ g) powdered cardamom

## OREGANO SPICE

*Add this sprinkle to chili, guacamole, salsa, cornbread, and dehydrated flax or nut crackers/ savory biscuits.*

1 tablespoon (6 g) powdered oregano

1 teaspoon (2 g) powdered coriander

1 teaspoon (2 g) powdered cumin

1 teaspoon (2 g) powdered paprika

1 teaspoon (2 g) powdered garlic

## PEPPERMILL BLEND

*The combination of these herbs adds a zest of flavor to your food. Use a large peppermill to grind these herbs, as the juniper berries can get stuck in a small one.*

2 tablespoons (12 g) whole black peppercorns

2 tablespoons (11 g) whole coriander

1 teaspoon (4 g) dried juniper berries

## RED POWDER

*I love this sprinkle on rice, and I apply it lavishly to egg dishes. It is full of vitamin C and cardiovascular tonic properties. This is a great addition to summer smoothies and green drinks.*

2 tablespoons (12 g) powdered rose hips

2 tablespoons (12 g) powdered hawthorn berry

1 tablespoon (6 g) powdered red rose petals

1 tablespoon (6 g) powdered orange peel

Dash of powdered clove

## SALAD SPRINKLE

*I make a quart (1 L) of this sprinkle at a time and can hardly keep the jar stocked. Mix this sprinkle into salads, rice, eggs, and steamed vegetables.*

2 tablespoons (50 g) whole sesame seeds

2 tablespoons (12 g) powdered chive

1 teaspoon (1 g) powdered seaweed (wakame or kombu)

¼ teaspoon (½ g) powdered black pepper

## SAVORY SEASONING

*Add this sprinkle to any savory dish that has an egg batter such as quiche, frittata, or omelets. Put on breakfast home-style potatoes and egg or tofu scrambles.*

3 tablespoons (18 g) powdered chives

2 tablespoons (10 g) powdered parsley

1 tablespoon (6 g) powdered rosemary

1 tablespoon (6 g) powdered oregano

2 teaspoons (3 g) powdered thyme

2 teaspoons (4 g) powdered garlic

1 teaspoon (1 g) powdered basil

1 teaspoon (2 g) powdered lavender

1 teaspoon (1 g) powdered bay leaf

1 teaspoon (2 g) powdered black pepper

## SOUP BOUQUET

*Put this mixture of dried, whole, or powdered herbs into a muslin pouch and soak in simmering soup broths.*

1 tablespoon (2 g) dried parsley

1 tablespoon (6 g) dried lemon balm

1 teaspoon (2 g) dried fennel seed

1 dried bay leaf

1 star anise pod

## SWEET AND SPICY HERB RUB

½ cup (120 g) dehydrated cane juice

2 tablespoons (12 g) powdered paprika

2 teaspoons (4 g) powdered black pepper

¼ teaspoon (½ g) powdered star anise

## TURMERIC-GINGER SPRINKLE

*These herbs are anti-inflammatory and can help soothe the symptoms of many ailments from allergies to arthritis. I put a dash of this on whatever is in my sandwich or pita pocket. Sprinkle it on lettuce wraps, casseroles, and salads. The warming qualities of these herbs make this the perfect sprinkle to coat winter meals.*

2 tablespoons (12 g) powdered turmeric

½ teaspoon (1 g) powdered ginger

### HERBAL SALT

Herbed salts are a combination of dried powdered herbs and salt. Herbed salts can be used instead of salt at mealtime, and they also make good rubs for tenderizing food before cooking or dehydrating.

## ALL-PURPOSE HERBED SALT

*This salt helps tenderize food, making it more digestible. Benefit from the therapeutic effect of the herbs while adding a gourmet flair to your food. Rub it on fish, vegetables, and meats.*

¼ cup (63 g) salt

2 tablespoons (12 g) powdered coriander

1 tablespoon (6 g) powdered turmeric

1 teaspoon (2 g) powdered cumin

1 teaspoon (2 g) powdered fennel seed

1 teaspoon (2 g) powdered mustard seed

½ teaspoon (1 g) powdered star anise

## CITRUS SALT

*Add olive oil and vinegar to this rub, spread it on your summer vegetables, and then grill them on the barbecue.*

2 tablespoons (30 g) salt

¼ cup (24 g) powdered orange peel

1 tablespoon (6 g) powdered black pepper

## HERB SALT

2 tablespoons (30 g) salt

2 tablespoons (12 g) powdered cumin

1 tablespoon (6 g) powdered oregano

1 tablespoon (4 g) powdered thyme

Dash of powdered cayenne

## MUSTARD-SALT RUB

*If you are having an uninspired day in the kitchen, pull out a couple of herbed salts and let them do the work of livening up your meals.*

¼ cup (63 g) salt

3 tablespoons (18 g) powdered mustard seed

2 teaspoons (3 g) powdered thyme

2 teaspoons (4 g) celery seed

½ teaspoon (½ g) powdered bay leaf

½ teaspoon (½ g) powdered allspice

## PAPRIKA-GARLIC SALT

*Enjoy this sprinkle on barbecued potatoes and squash. Put it on fish and vegetables before cooking. When I sprinkle my food, I think good thoughts about the people for whom I am cooking. Adding your thoughts to your food is another simple and powerful way to initiate healing in your everyday life.*

¼ cup (63 g) salt

¼ cup (24 g) powdered paprika

2 tablespoons (12 g) powdered garlic

1 tablespoon (6 g) powdered black pepper

1 teaspoon (1 g) powdered thyme

## ROSEMARY SALT

*Use this like salt at the table. Herbed salts also belong in the bathtub. Take time for yourself and put a cup of Rosemary Salt into your bathwater. I also like to add ¼ cup (60 ml) of olive oil to ½ cup (125 g) of Rosemary Salt, scrub it all over my body, and then rinse off in the shower.*

¼ cup (63 g) salt

¼ cup (24 g) powdered rosemary

1 teaspoon (2 g) celery seed

## SAVORY SALT RUB

½ cup (125 g) salt

3 tablespoons (15 g) powdered parsley

2 tablespoons (12 g) powdered oregano

2 tablespoons (12 g) powdered chives

1 tablespoon (6 g) powdered turmeric

1 teaspoon (1 g) powdered bay leaf

CHAPTER 13

# Herbal Kitchen Meals

One of the best ways to incorporate herbs into your meals is to make and use the oils, vinegars, pestos, and salts covered in the previous chapters. These condiments help you add a splash, dollop, or sprinkle of herbal goodness to anything on your plate. When you have these staples at the ready, you'll find they make their way into all kinds of foods, adding layers of delicious flavor. I always keep a couple of herbal infused oils and sprinkles on our kitchen table, to up the nutritional value and the flavor of almost every meal.

The recipes in this section are the ones that make it to the table on busy days after work and school and driving everyone where they need to go. They are the tried-and-true dishes, the ones that have nourished my family for years. They represent the real, honest food we eat. Simple, healthy, and full of herbs.

The recipes are organized by season to take advantage of what's available, but also to provide dishes that suit your body's needs at each time of year. We crave foods that temper the warming or cooling effects of each season: Heavier foods insulate the body in winter, while spring calls for lighter fare to help shed the weight of winter. Summer salads keep us cool and autumn roots keep us nourished and hydrated during that transitional season.

As a general rule, I always use organic ingredients and try to source them locally whenever possible. It's important to me that the ingredients I cook with are not only organic but are grown by people who care about sustainability.

Biodynamic farming meets the standards of organic farming, but it goes much further, requiring that farms set aside land for biodiversity and meet other earth-friendly criteria. If you can find biodynamically grown food, that's great. If you can't, don't stress. If ingredients are imported, try to look for Fair Trade Certified. Buying Fair Trade products ensures that the companies producing them put people and the planet first. Do the best you can; these are just guidelines.

## RECIPES FOR WINTER

Oregano Beet Hummus

Herby Meatballs

Curried Vegetable Dal

Herbed Rice Stuffed Bell Peppers

 ## OREGANO BEET HUMMUS

*When I look at a recipe, I immediately think, "Where can I add another layer of herbs?" Some recipes may call for only half a teaspoon of dried herbs, but I almost always at least double what the recipe calls for. If it calls for only dried herbs, I try to add fresh ones as well, even if it's just a garnish.*

*Some foods, like pesto, sauces, marinades, dressings, and rice are the perfect medium for adding herbs—they all lend themselves to adding layers of flavor. Hummus is another one of those great carrier foods.*

*This recipe is delicious as is but you can experiment with different combinations of veggies and herbs, such as roasted parsnips and oregano or scallions and parsley. The possibilities are endless. The ruby red color of this dip is gorgeous and it's a simple crowd-pleasing appetizer when served with sliced veggies. I also like to toss cooked greens with a small amount for a side dish.*

## INGREDIENTS

3 cups (800 g) cooked chick peas

2 medium-sized beets, roasted, peeled, and chopped

1 cup (250 ml) vegetable or bone broth

¼ cup (60 ml) fresh lemon juice

3 tablespoons (45 ml) olive oil

2 tablespoons (36 g) tahini

½ cup (15 g) chopped fresh parsley

¼ cup (8 g) chopped fresh oregano

2 cloves garlic, peeled

1 teaspoon (6 g) salt

Fresh oregano and parsley, for garnishing

Sliced vegetables such as carrots, celery, and cucumbers for serving.

## DIRECTIONS

1. Combine all the ingredients in the bowl of a food processor and blend until smooth.

2. Taste and add more garlic or lemon juice, if you like. You can also add a little water for a thinner consistency. Blend until smooth.

3. Garnish with fresh oregano and parsley and serve with sliced vegetables.

# HERBY MEATBALLS

*My husband is a meat and potatoes kind of guy. Me? Not so much. A few years ago, he took charge of cooking our meals three days a week. I had always been the primary cook for our family, so this shift was a big help to me, but when we sat down to dinner, I found myself asking, "Where's the veggies?"*

*Now don't get me wrong, I love my husband's meatloaf, chili, and mashed potatoes, but I don't want to eat meat and potatoes every day of the week. It's important to include vegetables on the plate at every meal. To help him understand, I talked to my husband about how the vegetables, herbs, and spices help your body digest meat and how important that is for not just our own health, but for our son's growing body. The result is this recipe, which packs a lot of vegetables into a family-friendly dish. It's one of those magical meals that satisfies everyone.*

## INGREDIENTS

1 lb. (450 g) ground turkey

½ cup (75 g) ground sunflower seeds

1 egg

1 teaspoon (5 ml) fresh lemon juice

1 clove garlic, minced

2 teaspoons (3 g) powdered coriander

1 teaspoon (1 g) paprika

1 teaspoon (1 g) powdered cumin

½ teaspoon (3 g) salt

3 tablespoons (45 ml) ghee

1 teaspoon (2 g) powdered cinnamon

½ teaspoon (1/2 g) powdered allspice

1 yellow onion, finely minced

1 celery stalk, finely minced

1 small carrot, finely grated

1 small parsnip, finely grated

¼ cup (8 g) minced fresh parsley

Chopped fresh mint and parsley, for garnishing

**DIRECTIONS**

1. In a large bowl, combine the turkey, ground sunflower seeds, egg, lemon juice, garlic, coriander, paprika, cumin, and salt. Mix well and set aside.

2. Warm 1 tablespoon (15 ml) of ghee in a skillet over low heat. Add the cinnamon and allspice and cook for 1 minute or until you begin to smell the spices, taking care not to burn them.

3. Add the onions, celery, and remaining 2 tablespoons (30 ml) of ghee. Cook until the onions are soft and translucent. Remove the pan from the heat and add the carrots and parsnips to the onions and mix well.

4. Add the vegetables to the bowl with the turkey and spices. Add the parsley and mix well.

5. Preheat the oven to 300°F (150°C). Roll the meatball mixture into small (2-in/50 mm) balls and place them on a baking sheet. Bake the meatballs for 30 to 40 minutes.

6. Garnish with chopped fresh mint and parsley.

 CURRIED VEGETABLE DAL

*I grew up eating cold cereal and milk for breakfast all year long. Since studying the wisdom of Ayurveda, I have learned that warm, easy to digest foods are the best winter breakfast. As the days grow colder and darker, your body starts to crave more insulating foods. Cold mornings call for replacing fruit and smoothies with warm, heartier breakfasts. This warm, well-spiced soup is the perfect way to start a winter day—it's deeply nourishing and helps prevent the cold from settling into your body.*

*It is always a good idea to add lots of herbs and spices to heavier meals, to help keep your blood moving and to fight off the congestion that winter can bring on.*

## INGREDIENTS

¼ cup (60 ml) coconut oil

1 cinnamon stick

6 green cardamom pods, cracked open

½ teaspoon (1 g) powdered cloves

1 onion, chopped

1 teaspoon (3 g) grated fresh ginger

2 bay leaves

1 teaspoon (2 g) powdered cumin

1 teaspoon (2 g) powdered fenugreek

1 teaspoon (2 g) powdered turmeric

2 tablespoons (14 g) powdered coriander

2 cups (500 ml) vegetable or bone broth

1 cup (240 g) red lentils

1 small head of cauliflower, cut into small florets

1 sweet potato, peeled and cubed

½ red bell pepper, chopped

1 cup (75 g) chopped fresh shiitake mushrooms

1-14 oz. (400 ml) can of coconut milk

## DIRECTIONS

1. Heat 2 tablespoons (24 g) of coconut oil in a soup pot over medium heat.

2. Add the cinnamon, cardamom, and cloves and heat for 2 minutes. Add the remaining 2 tablespoons (24 g) of coconut oil and sauté the onion for about 5 minutes or until golden.

3. Add the ginger and the bay leaves and sauté for 1 minute. Reduce the heat to low and add the cumin, fenugreek, turmeric, and coriander. Sauté for 2 minutes. Add the stock and the lentils and bring to a gentle simmer. Cook for 15 minutes.

4. Add the cauliflower, sweet potato, red pepper, and mushrooms and simmer for an additional 10 minutes. Add the coconut milk and simmer an additional 5 minutes, until the lentils are soft but not mushy.

# HERB RICE STUFFED BELL PEPPERS

*My grandfather was an avid, lifelong fisherman and my dad was an ocean diver. Growing up, we had large freezers stocked with the ocean's harvest along with wild and farmed foods that my dad and grandpa traded fish for.*

*Every summer we swapped fish for bell peppers with a local farmer. What does one do with boxes of bell peppers? Make stuffed peppers, of course, and store them in the freezer to eat all winter long. Once a week throughout the winter we'd wake up to a pan of stuffed peppers defrosting on the counter. It was a seasonal staple in our house. Over the years I've added a lot more spice and veggies to the filling and have upgraded the topping from ketchup to fresh herbs.*

*This dish was not on the original list of recipes I wanted to share with you. I thought to myself, "Everyone knows this recipe; there is nothing new here." However, I realized just how important this dish has been to shaping how I think about food and culinary culture. How we traded for the bell peppers, how we fed our family, is a way of being that was embedded into my cells: The earth is incredibly abundant. Take care of the harvest you receive, no matter how big it is. Share what you have.*

## INGREDIENTS

1 lb. (450 g) ground beef

3 tablespoons (8 g) minced fresh savory

3 tablespoons (8 g) minced fresh thyme

10 red bell peppers

1½ cups (275 g) rice

½ cup (120 g) small sized, split yellow lentils

4 cups (1 L) vegetable or bone broth

2 bay leaves

1 large yellow onion, diced

2 celery stalks, diced

1 cup (75 g) chopped mushrooms

2 cloves garlic, minced

1 tablespoon (6 g) paprika

1 tablespoon (3 g) dried thyme

2 teaspoons (12 g) tamarind paste

½ teaspoon (1 g) cayenne

1 teaspoon (6 g) salt

1 tablespoon (15 ml) olive oil

¼ cup (60 ml) red wine

12 oz. (340 g) can chunky tomato sauce (or 2-3 fresh tomatoes, chopped)

1 cup (250 ml) vegetable or bone broth

2 scallions, sliced

Chopped fresh parsley, for garnishing

## DIRECTIONS

1. Combine the ground beef, fresh savory, and thyme in a bowl and mix well. Cover and refrigerate while you prepare the other ingredients.

2. Cut the tops off of the bell peppers and discard the stems. Chop the tops and set aside. Scrape the seeds and membranes out from inside the peppers and discard.

3. Fill a large pot halfway with water and bring to a boil. Boil the peppers for 8 minutes, remove them, and set them aside. Discard the cooking water.

4. Combine the rice, lentils, broth, and bay leaf in a medium-sized pot and bring to a boil. Reduce the heat to low, cover, and simmer 25 minutes or until the rice is tender.

5. Combine the onions, chopped pepper tops, celery, mushrooms, and ¼ cup (60 ml) water or broth in a large skillet and simmer over medium heat until the liquid has evaporated. Add the garlic and sauté for one minute.

6. Move the vegetables to one side of the pan and in the open space, add the paprika, thyme, tamarind paste, cayenne, salt, and olive oil and cook for 1 minute. Add the red wine to de-glaze the pan, scraping up any bits that have stuck to the bottom, and then mix everything together.

7. Add the ground beef and break it up in the pan, cooking it until it's no longer pink. Add the cooked rice and tomato sauce and mix everything together.

8. Fill the bell peppers with the rice and beef mixture and place them in a baking pan. Add 1 cup (250 ml) of vegetable or bone broth to the pan and bake at 350°F (177°C) for 30 minutes.

9. Serve garnished with scallions and fresh parsley. For extra flavor, drizzle with Paprika Oil (see page 213).

# RECIPES FOR SPRING

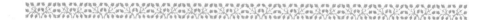

Herbed Egg Muffins with Mint Sauce

Best Potluck Quinoa

Asparagus with Chives

Quick and Easy Miso Soup

## HERBED EGG MUFFINS WITH MINT SAUCE

*I don't like to eat breakfast until about ten but my husband, Michael, and my son wake up hungry. Michael has taken on more of the cooking for our family, including breakfast. He'll joke with me and say, "Hey Kami, look, I added some greens to the eggs." And when I make breakfast I say, "Hey look, I put some eggs in with the greens."*

*Every herbalist has a favorite egg recipe because it's another great place to increase the herbal quotient. You can customize the egg muffins: Pack the muffin well to the top with the greens and add in just enough egg to hold them together, or fill them half full of greens and then add the egg.*

*This recipe evolves constantly depending on what greens the garden provides. I like to decorate the top of the muffins with a cherry tomato, a basil or sage leaf, or a calendula blossom before putting them into the oven.*

## HERBED EGG MUFFINS INGREDIENTS

1 leek, white and light green parts only, finely chopped

1½ cups (115 g) chopped shiitake mushrooms

¼ cup (60 ml) water

1 clove garlic, minced

½ teaspoon (3 g) salt

2 cups (60 g) greens, finely chopped (chard, kale, dandelion, spinach, sorrel, or lamb's quarter)

½ cup (15 g) chopped parsley

1 tablespoon (3 g) minced fresh marjoram

1 tablespoon (3 g) minced fresh rosemary

1 tablespoon (3 g) minced fresh garlic chives

1 tablespoon (3 g) minced fresh basil

8 eggs

½ teaspoon (1 g) powdered nutmeg

4 tablespoons (60 ml) ghee

Mint Sauce, for garnish

## DIRECTIONS

1. Heat a skillet over medium heat. Add the leek, mushrooms, and water and cook until the water has evaporated and the leeks are soft (about 4 minutes). Add the garlic and salt and remove from the heat.

2. Add the greens, parsley, and the aromatic herbs to the cooked leeks and mushrooms. Mix well. The warmth of the leeks and mushrooms will wilt the greens. Set aside.

3. Combine the eggs and the nutmeg in a bowl. Beat the eggs for 1 minute, until frothy.

4. Preheat the oven to 350ºF (177ºC). Grease a muffin pan generously with ghee.

5. Divide the greens among the muffin wells and then pour the eggs over the top. Bake for about 20 minutes, or until the eggs are set. Remove the muffins from the pan and serve with Mint Sauce or one of the pestos from chapter 11.

## MINT SAUCE INGREDIENTS

½ small jalapeno pepper, sliced in half and de-seeded

1 cup (45 g) fresh mint leaves, chopped

½ cup (125 ml) water

½ cup (30 g) dried, shredded coconut

½ teaspoon (3 g) salt

¼ cup (60 ml) fresh lime juice

1 teaspoon (5 g) ghee

½ teaspoon (2 g) black mustard seed

½ teaspoon (1 g) cumin seed

## DIRECTIONS

1. Combine the jalapeno, mint, water, coconut, salt, and lime juice in the bowl of a food processor and blend into a smooth paste. Scrape the paste into a bowl or a jar.

2. Heat the ghee in a small skillet over medium heat. Add the mustard and cumin seeds, cover, and heat until they begin to pop. Remove the skillet from the heat. When the seeds are cool, add them to the mint paste with the water and mix well.

3. If possible, let the flavors blend for a couple of hours before serving.

# BEST POTLUCK QUINOA

*Quinoa is the perfect grain for spring. It is a complete protein, yet it's light and lends itself well to all kinds of vegetables and spices. I like to cook it with seaweed for an added dose of nutrition.*

*One of the keys to this dish is chopping the vegetables as finely as you can. Quinoa is soft and fluffy and if you mix it with large crunchy vegetables, the variation between textures is not so great. Challenge yourself to see just how small you can chop the green beans and jicama.*

*This dish makes a great contribution to a potluck dinner. For one such dinner, I decided to marinate some goat cheese in Indulgence Oil (page 211) overnight and then sprinkled the marinated cheese and oil onto the quinoa salad. The flavor heavens parted, and the salad went from good to over the top.*

*At the potluck, a woman came up to me and said, "I heard you made the quinoa salad. I've got to have that recipe! My husband won't eat quinoa, but he said this salad was so good that he wanted to know how to make it. Can you please give me the recipe?" I knew I had a winner.*

## INGREDIENTS

1 cup (170 g) uncooked quinoa

2-in (5-cm) piece of kombu or wakame seaweed (optional)

2 cups (500 ml) vegetable or bone broth

2–3 (30–45 ml) tablespoons olive oil

2 tablespoons (30 ml) fresh lemon juice

1 teaspoon (2 g) paprika

1 teaspoon (2 g) powdered coriander

¼ teaspoon (1/2 g) powdered cumin

½ teaspoon (3 g) salt

1 cup (150 g) finely chopped green beans

½ cup (75 g) finely chopped jicama

1 cup (30 g) minced chard

1 carrot, finely grated

3 tablespoons (30 g) dried currants

3 tablespoons (6 g) fresh minced parsley

2 scallions, finely chopped

Zest from 1 lemon

Marinated Goat Cheese:

    6 oz (170 g) goat cheese

    3 tablespoons (20 ml) Indulgence Oil (page 211)

**DIRECTIONS**

1. Combine the quinoa, seaweed, and broth in a pot and bring to a boil. Reduce heat to low and simmer, uncovered, for 10 to 15 minutes, until all the liquid is absorbed. Remove and discard the seaweed, cover, and set aside for 5 minutes, then fluff with a fork. Scrape the quinoa into a large bowl and set aside to cool.

2. Add the olive oil, lemon juice, spices, and salt to the cooked quinoa and mix well. Add the remaining ingredients, cover, and refrigerate for a couple of hours before serving.

3. For extra flavor, marinate the goat cheese in the Indulgence Oil in the refrigerator for a couple of hours.

4. To serve, scatter the marinated cheese on top of the salad and drizzle with the remaining oil.

 ASPARAGUS WITH CHIVES

*One of the joys of spring is that asparagus, my favorite vegetable, is in season. If you have breakfast or dinner at my house in March, I will most likely serve asparagus. For about two months, it is the main vegetable on our table, then it goes out of season and we have to wait until next spring!*

*This plate of yum takes less than ten minutes to make and it will be one of the first things to be eaten up. Make the dressing in advance if you can. The chives will have time to infuse the oil and vinegar, adding more flavor. This recipe yields more dressing than you need for one bunch of asparagus but you'll have some left over for a salad or cooked greens.*

**INGREDIENTS**

1 lb. (450 g) asparagus

**Dressing**

1 cup (250 ml) olive oil

¼ cup (60 ml) balsamic vinegar

3 teaspoons (15 ml) maple syrup

1 garlic clove, minced

¼ cup (12 g) minced fresh chives

½ teaspoon (3 g) salt

**Garnish**

¼ cup (60 g) sesame seeds

Zest of 1 orange

**DIRECTIONS**

1. Steam the asparagus until tender crisp.
2. To make the dressing, whisk all the ingredients together in a small bowl.
3. Drizzle the cooked asparagus with ½ cup (120 ml) of the dressing just before serving. Garnish with sesame seeds and orange zest.

## QUICK AND EASY MISO SOUP

*You may think of miso soup as a staple on a Japanese table, but this simple, delicious soup is also a perfect breakfast food. It's full of protein, vitamins, minerals, and hydrating electrolytes—it's nutritious and satisfying yet doesn't require a lot of digestive energy. If you aren't used to eating soup for breakfast, try it! This is what I eat when I write, so that my brain can stay focused on my work.*

*This recipe yields a small batch as the soup is best consumed fresh. A dollop of the Zesty Pesto from chapter 11 makes a delicious topping.*

**INGREDIENTS**

2 cups (500 ml) water, vegetable, or bone broth

1 teaspoon (3 g) finely grated ginger

1 teaspoon (3 g) hijiki seaweed (or your favorite seaweed)

1 cup (125 g) of chopped vegetables (zucchini, cabbage, and bok choy)

1 scallion, chopped

1 tablespoon (9 g) grated daikon radish

3 tablespoons (51 g) miso

**DIRECTIONS**

1. Combine the water, vegetable or bone broth, ginger, and seaweed in a pot and bring to a simmer.

2. Add the chopped vegetables, scallions, and daikon radish and simmer until the vegetables are soft, about 8 minutes. Remove from the heat and set aside to cool for a few minutes.

3. Scoop the miso into a small bowl, add a spoonful or two of broth, and mash into a paste. Add to the soup, stir, and serve.

# RECEIPES FOR SUMMER

Fennel Chicken Salad

Green Garden Soup

Mom's Summer Salad

The Best Barley Salad

## FENNEL CHICKEN SALAD

*You can create a delicious summer meal by wrapping this crunchy chicken salad and a hand-ful of fresh herbs and sprouts into lettuce or kale leaves. The leafy greens, juicy fennel root, and cooling cilantro are the perfect antidote to summer's heat.*

### INGREDIENTS

**Salad**

3 cups (420 g) cooked, shredded chicken

3 cups (267 g) shredded Napa cabbage

1 cup (89 g) shredded red cabbage

1 cup (89 g) shredded fennel root

¼ cup (15 g) minced fresh parsley

¼ cup (15 g) chopped cilantro

2 scallions, finely chopped

3 tablespoons (28 g) finely grated fresh burdock root

2 teaspoons (4 g) celery seed

1 teaspoon (2 g) black pepper

**Dressing**

⅓ cup (80 ml) apple cider vinegar

⅓ cup (80 ml) olive oil

2–3 tablespoons (44–70 ml) honey

3 teaspoons (9 g) lemon zest

1 teaspoon (2 g) powdered juniper berry

½ teaspoon (3 g) salt

Lettuce, kale, or cabbage leaves, for serving

Salad Sprinkle (see chapter 12), for garnishing

Fresh herbs such as parsley, cilantro, mint, and bean sprouts, for garnishing

### DIRECTIONS

1. Combine the salad ingredients in a bowl and mix well. Refrigerate until ready to serve.

2. To make the dressing, combine all the ingredients in a small bowl or a jar and mix well.

3. To serve, drizzle the dressing over the salad and mix well. Serve with lettuce, kale, or cabbage leaves, Salad Sprinkle, fresh herbs, and bean sprouts.

 GREEN GARDEN SOUP

*The Good Earth Natural Food Store has been providing my community with superb organic food for more than forty-five years and serves the best homemade lunch around. Their Green River Soup hasn't been on the menu for years now, but I have recreated it at home. It's a hydrating, satisfying meal for a hot summer day, when you don't feel like eating, but you need nourishment.*

*You can use any greens you like–chard, spinach, kale, bok choy, watercress. I happen to love a combination of spinach and watercress; but use whatever is in peak season or you have on hand.*

*I confess, I have never made this soup the same way twice, but it's delicious every time!*

**INGREDIENTS**

3 tablespoons (30 g) cashews, soaked overnight

1 cup (250 ml) water

2 cups (60 g) fresh greens

2 cups (312 g) peeled, chopped cucumber

1 cup (160 g) green peas

1 cup (125 g) chopped zucchini

1 cup (30 g) cilantro, chopped

2 celery stalks, chopped

Handful of chopped fresh basil

Handful of dandelion leaf (or more, depending on your taste preference)

¼ cup (40 g) hemp seeds

2 tablespoons (30 ml) lime juice

2 teaspoons (2 g) dulse flakes

½ teaspoon (1 g) cumin

½ teaspoon (3 g) salt

Combine all the ingredients in a food processer and blend until creamy.

## MOM'S SUMMER SALAD

*Growing up, near Yolo County, California, the largest exporter of tomatoes in the United States, we rarely ate tomatoes from the store. When I was little, my mom worked in the tomato fields during the harvest. One of my earliest plant memories is playing in the fields with my little brother, with the plants towering over us. We ate SO many tomatoes. To this day, when I smell a tomato plant I am instantly transported to the memory of playing in those fields.*

*Once the tomatoes were ripe, my mom made this salad almost every day. Fresh tomatoes, cucumber, and red onion were a staple on our table all summer long. It's a simple recipe using ingredients that were made for each other. I added the fresh basil and calendula petals when I started making it for my family.*

*There is something special that happens around your family table: The combination of flavors, aromas, and feelings add up to something hard to describe, but soul-satisfying, and you are deeply nourished.*

**INGREDIENTS**

1 large cucumber, thinly sliced

2 tomatoes, sliced

½ red onion, thinly sliced

½ cup (120 ml) olive oil

¼ cup (60 ml) red wine vinegar

½ cup (15 g) basil, chopped

3 tablespoons (3 g) fresh parsley, minced

1 tablespoon (6 g) fresh thyme or 1 teaspoon (½ g) dried thyme

Salt and pepper to taste

Handful of fresh calendula petals

**DIRECTIONS**

Arrange the sliced vegetables on a plate and drizzle the olive oil and red wine vinegar over them. Sprinkle with the fresh herbs and salt and pepper and garnish with the calendula petals.

 THE BEST BARLEY SALAD

*We live in a county where there are lots of organic farms and you can find a farm-to-table celebration on pretty much any weekend in the summer. I love getting to know the people who grow our food, so you'll often find me out in a field or at one of these dinners.*

*It was at one of these dinners that I had this barley salad. By now you realize that if I taste something I love, I instantly start thinking about how I might make it at home. I sat down on a hay bale, studied the salad, and tried to figure out the ingredients so I could recreate it. When*

*it looked like he had a spare moment, I went over to the chef and said, "Wow, BEST barley salad ever . . . red onion, paprika, garlic, cumin, oregano, mint, and, what am I missing?" He was pretty busy, cooking for everyone. He said, "Thanks, let's see, it's also got some lime juice and onion powder."*

*I came home and started working on recreating the best barley salad. I worked on it for a while and came up with this rendition, which I think lives up to its name. What do you think?*

## INGREDIENTS

3 cups (200 g) cooked barley
1 cup (150 g) red onion, finely minced
1 cup (30 g) minced fresh parsley
Handful of fresh mint, minced

### Dressing

¼ cup (60 ml) olive oil
4 teaspoons (20 ml) red wine vinegar
1 teaspoon (5 ml) lime juice
1 clove garlic, minced
2 teaspoons (3 g) paprika
1 teaspoon (1 g) dried oregano
1 teaspoon (2 g) onion powder
½ teaspoon (3 g) salt
¼ teaspoon (1/2 g) cumin

1 firm avocado, chopped

## DIRECTIONS

1. Combine the barley, onion, parsley, and mint in a bowl.
2. To make the dressing, combine all the ingredients in a small bowl and mix well. Pour the dressing over the salad and mix well.
3. Add the chopped avocado just before serving.

# RECITES FOR FALL

Sunchokes with Anise Hyssop

Alchemical Autumn Veggies

Garlic Parsnip Mash with Rosemary Butter

Kashke Bademjan

 ## SUNCHOKES WITH ANISE HYSSOP

*When I first started studying herbal medicine, I spent a year as a garden apprentice working full time at what is now the Occidental Arts and Ecology Center in Northern California. One afternoon in early fall, after harvesting a big bunch of sunchokes, I went to the garden to forage for dinner, thinking I would pick some thyme and maybe the very last of the basil. The basil was looking a little scraggly, but the anise hyssop was at its peak. The vibrant purple flowers were so alive they were calling to me! I had only used anise hyssop for tea and desserts and never thought of using it in a main dish, but I was determined to try. It turns out that the sweet, fruity flavor of anise hyssop goes perfectly with sunchokes. Thus, a match was made in the garden that I had to bring to the table.*

*If you can't find anise hyssop, you can use lemon balm. It, too, has a sweet, pungent flavor that compliments the mild sunchokes. My secret wish is that you'll be inspired to grow your own anise hyssop and Jerusalem artichokes and make your own matches in the garden.*

### INGREDIENTS
1 lb. (450 g) sunchokes (also known as Jerusalem artichokes)
1 cup (250 ml) water or broth

**Garnish**

Butter

½ cup (15 g) fresh anise hyssop or lemon balm leaves, minced

Lemon wedges

Salt, to taste

Handful of pumpkin seeds, roasted

## DIRECTIONS

1. Steam the sunchokes in a pot with water or broth until they are soft, about 15 minutes.

2. Garnish with butter, fresh anise hyssop or lemon balm leaves, lemon, salt, and pumpkin seeds.

## ALCHEMICAL AUTUMN VEGGIES

*Roasting vegetables is a technique that takes little effort, but yields flavorful results. All you have to do is chop up the veggies, put them on a pan, throw them in a warm oven, and you're done. The trick to this dish is cutting the squash and other vegetables in such a way that they cook evenly, together. This is something that you learn over time. For example, carrots cook quicker than rutabaga, so cut the carrot a little bigger than the rutabaga.*

*Alchemy Oil is one of those oils I always have on hand. You can drizzle it on potatoes, winter squash, rice, or scrambled eggs. Or you can add vinegar and turn it into a salad dressing.*

## INGREDIENTS

4 cups (800 g) peeled and chopped root vegetables, such as carrots, rutabagas, turnips, onions, parsnips, celery root

1 cup (200 g) peeled and cubed winter squash

½ cup (125 ml) water

**Garnish**

Alchemy Oil (Chapter 9)

Handful of fresh arugula/rocket

Salt

**DIRECTIONS**

1. Preheat the oven to 350 degrees (177°C).

2. Spread the chopped veggies and squash on a sheet pan and add the water to the pan.

3. Bake for 30 minutes or until the vegetables are tender, but not overcooked.

4. Drizzle Alchemy Oil over the vegetables and garnish with fresh arugula and salt.

## GARLIC PARSNIP MASH

*As the leaves begin to drop, the dry winds of autumn can kick up tension and irritability in the body. The changing weather pattern calls for dishes that help us feel calm and grounded. Garlic Parsnip Mash fits that bill. The sweet root vegetables and healthy fat make this dish nourishing, and it's delicious and super easy to make.*

*My dad was a great gardener. One year he planted a few too many parsnip plants and that fall he brought me two large boxes of them. This recipe, like the Herb Rice Stuffed Bell Peppers (page 256–258), was born out of abundance. My dad loved the harvest. He loved preserving, storing, and putting food on the table. Thanks Dad.*

**INGREDIENTS**

2 cups (400 g) peeled and chopped parsnips

2 cups (400 g) peeled and chopped sweet potato

2½ cups (625 ml) vegetable or bone broth

2 bay leaves

2 cloves garlic, minced

½ teaspoon (3 g) salt

Savory Sauté Ghee (chapter 10)

Fresh calendula petals, for garnishing

**DIRECTIONS**

1. Combine the parsnips, potatoes, broth, and bay leaf in a pot and cook until the vegetables are soft, about 30 minutes.

2. Drain the liquid, remove the bay leaves, and mash the parsnips and potatoes. Add the garlic and salt.

3. Drizzle Savory Sauté Ghee or your favorite herbal ghee on the mash and serve garnished with the fresh calendula petals.

## KASHKE BADEMJAN

*I lived in San Francisco for many years and the wonderful thing about that city is that you meet people from all over the world. It was there that I became friends with Soheila and her family from Iran. She taught me how to drink tea with rose petals, henna my hair, take apart a pomegranate at record speed, brush my teeth with medicinal sticks, dine Persian style (sitting on the floor in a circle), and make kashke bademjan or Persian Eggplant Dip.*

*Making the kashke (whey), is an extra step and takes a little time, but is well worth the effort. You'll find recipes that call for just adding yogurt at the end, but I love the traditional method of cooking the kashke with the eggplant. Make sure you save some for leftovers because it tastes even better the next day.*

*I love this dish. I could eat it every day during eggplant season. From Soheila's Persian table through my kitchen with love to you.*

**INGREDIENTS**

2 cups (500 g) whole milk plain yogurt

5 large eggplants

½ cup (120 ml) water

1 large yellow onion, finely diced

¼ cup (60 ml) olive oil

2–4 cloves garlic, minced

1 teaspoon (6 g) salt

1 tablespoon (6 g) ground turmeric

3 tablespoons (6 g) dried peppermint

Pita bread, for serving

## DIRECTIONS

1. Line a strainer with cotton muslin and set it over a bowl. Put the yogurt in the strainer and set aside to drain for about 30 minutes. You should end up with ½ cup (125 ml) of whey, or kashke, that will have strained through the muslin.

2. Preheat the oven to 350 degrees (177°C). Cut the eggplants in half and place them cut side down on a sheet pan. Pour ¼ cup (60 ml) of water in the pan and bake for 20 minutes. Rotate the eggplants on the sheet to prevent them from sticking and bake for an additional 5 minutes, or until soft. Set aside to cool.

3. Once the eggplant is cool, scoop the flesh into a strainer and set aside to drain. Discard the skin.

4. Combine the diced onion and ¼ cup (60 ml) of water in a pan over medium-high heat. Sauté until the water has evaporated. Add 3 tablespoons (45 ml) of olive oil and continue to cook until golden brown. Add the garlic, ½ teaspoon (3 g) salt, turmeric, 2 tablespoons (4 g) of the dried mint, and sauté for 1 minute. Add the eggplant, whey, or kashke, reduce the heat to medium, and cook for about 10 minutes, stirring occasionally.

5. Heat the remaining tablespoon (15 ml) of olive oil in a small pan over medium heat. Add the remaining tablespoon (2 g) of dried mint and sauté for 1 minute, or until fragrant.

6. Combine the sautéed mint with 1 cup (285 g) of strained yogurt in a small bowl and mix well.

7. Serve the eggplant topped with dollops of mint yogurt and with pita bread or chopped veggies for dipping.

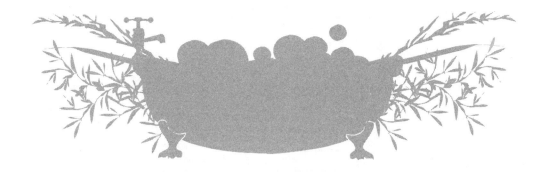

CHAPTER 14

# Herbal Baths and Foot Soaks

Immersing my entire body into a tub full of herbs is one of my favorite ways to use herbs. My skin is absorbing the herbal constituents, I am inhaling the medicine through the steam, and I get to lie in my bathtub. I experience so much pleasure as I smell the herbs and see the beautiful colors of the floating flowers and leaves. As I relax in the tub, my body is open to receiving the healing benefits of the herbs. Bathing with herbs is a significant component of my wellness program.

If you don't feel like soaking your entire body in a tub of tea, you can luxuriate with a foot soak instead. Steeping your feet in herbal tea is an enjoyable way to care for your body. Foot soaks are a feast for the feet. Immerse the multitudes of nerve endings in your feet in a tub of herbal tea, and let the herbs work you over. It is the treatment of least effort yet the effects are impressive. Get into the habit of making a foot soak for yourself anytime you feel a little out of sorts on any level.

# MAKING HERBAL BATHS

### METHOD #1: LOOSE HERB TEA BATH

Water

Large pot

Fresh or dried herbs

Strainer

1. Put 8 quarts (8 L) water into a large pot.
2. Add 2 cups (96 to 192 g) fresh herbs or 2 cups (36 to 192 g) dried herbs per 4 quarts (4 L) water.
3. Bring water and herbs to a boil, turn off the heat, and let herbs infuse for one hour.
4. Strain the herbs from the water, or leave them in the water if you want the herbs poured into the bathtub.
5. Reheat tea.
6. Pour strained or unstrained tea into drawn bathwater. You can strain out the herbs before you put the tea into the tub, or pour the herbs directly into the bathwater along with your tea. If you do not strain out the herbs, make sure you feel like cleaning up after your bath unless you do not mind a stained bathtub. (I have solved this problem by setting up an outdoor bathtub. I can stain the tub, I don't have to clean it out right after bathing, and I can lie in the fragrance of lavender flowers and rose petals under the stars and the full moon.)

### METHOD #2: TEA BAG BATH

I like to use dried herbs and make up ten tea bath bags at a time so I don't have to make one up at every bath time. Tie dried herbs into a little pouch of muslin and keep them in a container in the bathroom so they are ready to go when the bathwater is being drawn. Method #2 is a quicker way to make an herbal bath, but the therapeutic effects of the herbs are not as strong as adding a tea as described in Method #1.

Fresh or dried herbs

Cotton cloth, such as T-shirt fabric or muslin

Rubber band or string

1. Put ½ to 1 cup (36 to 96 g) of fresh herbs or ½ to 1 cup (8 to 96 g) dried herbs into a sock or a 7-by-7-inch (18-by-18-cm) piece of cotton fabric. If you use fresh herbs, the pouch needs to be used in the bathtub that day, or the herbs will mold.

2. Tie the string around the opening of the fabric so that the herbs are contained in the fabric pouch.

3. Hook the little sachet of herbs under the tub spout so the water will pour through the herbs as it goes into your bathtub. Once your bath is drawn, just let the bag of herbs float in the tub. Discard the herbs when you are done.

## METHOD #3: GARDEN BATH

Fresh herbs from the garden

I walk through the garden and pick several handfuls of whatever medicinal herbs are available and put them directly into the bathtub. What goes into the garden bath varies depending on the time of the year. Sometimes one herb is just dripping off the vine into my basket, and other times picking a little of everything that is in bloom is the way to go. Herbs that can be found in my garden baths are basil, calendula, California poppy, chamomile, chickweed, cypress, dandelion, elder flower, fennel seed, eucalyptus leaves, juniper berries, lavender, lemon balm, lemon verbena, mugwort, peppermint, pine needles, oak leaves, parsley, plantain, redwood needles, rose geranium, rosemary, rose petals, sage, spearmint, thyme, and yarrow. I just mush up the herbs in my hands and throw them into the tub. I love this part of my life.

# MAKING AN HERBAL FOOT SOAK

1.  Put 4 quarts (4 L) water into a large pot.

2.  Put up to 1 cup (48 to 96 g) fresh herbs or 1 cup (16 to 96 g) dried herbs into the pot.

3.  Bring water and herbs to a boil, turn off the heat, and let herbs infuse for one hour.

4.  Leave herbs in the water for the foot bath or strain them out. I like to leave the herbs in, as they continue to infuse the water, and I enjoy their color and texture.

5.  Reheat tea.

6.  Pour strained or unstrained tea into a foot basin.

7.  Soak your feet for ten minutes or for as long as you like. It isn't much of a mess to clean up; when you are finished, just pour the water and herbs into a garden bed outside.

# RECIPES

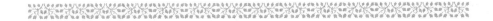

Any of the following recipes can be adapted to either a bath or a foot soak.

## ALIVE AND REVIVE BATH

*This bath helps with transitioning from one part of the day to another. After a full work-day, refresh yourself in this reviving blend of herbs and watch yourself come alive for an evening outing.*

8 quarts (8 L) water

1 cup (192 g) fresh whole juniper berries or 1 cup (80 g) dried juniper berries

½ cup (24 g) fresh rosemary or ½ cup (26 g) dried rosemary

½ cup (36 g) fresh calendula or ½ cup (8 g) dried calendula

2-inch (5-cm) piece fresh ginger

At Ease Foot Soak

4 quarts (4 L) water

¼ cup (24 g) fresh orange peel or ¼ cup (16 g) dried orange peel

¼ cup (18 g) fresh lavender or ¼ cup (4 g) dried lavender

¼ cup (24 g) fresh sage leaves or ¼ cup (24 g) dried sage leaves

¼ cup (28 g) fennel seed

## COOL-ME-DOWN FOOT SOAK

*If you are overheated or feel a headache coming on, make this foot soak. Let it cool down, immerse your feet in it, and feel the heat subside.*

4 quarts (4 L) water

¼ cup (8 g) fresh rose petals or ¼ cup (24 g) dried rose petals

2 tablespoons (12 g) fresh lemon balm or 2 tablespoons (12 g) dried lemon balm

1 tablespoon (3 g) fresh peppermint leaves or 1 tablespoon (6 g) dried peppermint
  leaves

## EMOTIONAL RESCUE BATH

*Herbal bathing can help you to relax and shift your state of mind.*

12 quarts (12 L) water

1 cup (96 g) fresh lemon balm or 1 cup (96 g) dried lemon balm

1 cup (30 g) fresh lemon verbena or 1 cup (96 g) dried lemon verbena

½ cup (36 g) fresh rose geranium or ½ cup (8 g) dried rose geranium

½ cup (36 g) fresh chamomile or ½ cup (8 g) dried chamomile

½ cup (15 g) fresh rose petals or ½ cup (48 g) dried rose petals

## FLOWER POWER BATH

*Flowers are healing. Their beauty, texture, and fragrance capture the senses, calm the mind, and ease the body. We all need rituals to help bring us back to ourselves. Stress, work, and excess stimulation keep the mind activated and can have a numbing effect on the body and emotions. Herbal bathing can be a healing meditation. Try this simple and easy way to let go. The water and herbs bring you back to your breath and to your senses, guiding you to feel and hear what is deep inside of you.*

8 quarts (8 L) water

1 cup (30 g) fresh rose petals or 1 cup (96 g) dried rose petals

½ cup (36 g) fresh calendula or ½ cup (8 g) dried calendula

½ cup (40 g) fresh elder flowers or ½ cup (8 g) dried elder flowers

½ cup (36 g) fresh chamomile or ½ cup (8 g) dried chamomile

## GENTLE DETOX BATH TEA

*Let the herbs help your body do its job of letting go of what it no longer needs.*

8 quarts (8 L) water

1 cup (30 g) fresh basil leaves or 1 cup (96 g) dried basil leaves

½ cup (59 g) fresh burdock pieces or ½ cup (96 g) dried burdock

¼ cup (30 g) sliced fresh ginger

## HEALING SKIN BATH TEA

*This bath helps with skin irritation such as acne, rashes, red splotches, and minor cuts.*

4 gallons (16 L) water

½ cup (36 g) fresh chamomile or ½ cup (8 g) dried chamomile

½ cup (40 g) fresh elder flowers or ½ cup (8 g) dried elder flowers

¼ cup (18 g) fresh lavender or ¼ cup (4 g) dried lavender

¼ cup (24 g) fresh lemon balm or ¼ cup (24 g) dried lemon balm

¼ cup (18 g) fresh rose geranium or ¼ cup (8 g) dried rose geranium

¼ cup (8 g) fresh rose petals or ¼ cup (24 g) dried rose petals

## INVIGORATING BATH

*Make a hot tea with these ingredients, pour it into your bath water, and feel the workday wash away.*

8 quarts (8 L) water

½ cup (24 g) fresh peppermint leaves or ½ cup (48 g) dried peppermint leaves

½ cup (36 g) fresh calendula or ½ cup (8 g) dried calendula

½ cup (24 g) fresh rosemary or ½ cup (26 g) dried rosemary

¼ cup (48 g) fresh juniper berries or ¼ cup (20 g) dried juniper berries

## LOVE YOUR LIFE HEALING BATH

*If a couple of weeks pass by and I haven't made the time to take an herbal bath, it is a sure sign that things are getting out of balance in my life. As a mom, it is easy for me to just stay focused on all the daily details required to care for everyone. Herbal bathing is one of the absolute necessities in my life. It is one of the primary ways I nourish and care for myself so that I can remain strong for others.*

4 gallons (16 L) water

1 cup (30 g) fresh mugwort or 1 cup (48 g) dried mugwort

1 cup (72 g) fresh calendula or 1 cup (16 g) dried calendula

1 cup (72 g) fresh lavender or 1 cup (16 g) dried lavender

½ cup (36 g) fresh rose geranium or ½ cup (8 g) dried rose geranium

## MOVE IT FOOT SOAK

*Increase circulation and warmth throughout your body with this foot soak.*

4 quarts (4 L) water

½ cup (48 g) fresh orange peel pieces or ½ cup (32 g) dried orange peel pieces

2 tablespoons (14 g) cinnamon stick pieces

2 tablespoons (15 g) fresh sliced ginger

## MUSCLE EASE BATH TEA

*If you have achy muscles, take some time to luxuriate in this aromatic bath.*

8 quarts (8 L) water

1 cup (30 g) fresh mugwort or 1 cup (24 g) dried mugwort

1 cup (48 g) fresh rosemary or 1 cup (52 g) dried rosemary leaves

¼ cup (8 g) fresh bay leaves or ¼ cup (12 g) dried bay leaves

¼ cup (30 g) fresh sliced ginger

## NO ITCH BATH TEA

*This bath will soothe and cool your skin.*

1 cup (90 g) rolled oats

1 cup (250 g) Epsom salt

½ cup (8 g) dried chamomile

¼ cup (4 g) dried lavender

¼ cup (24 g) dried rose petals

> Put the ingredients into a cloth pouch. Run the bathwater through the pouch, and then leave the pouch in the water as you bathe.

## REJUVENATION BATH TEA

8 quarts (8 L) water

2 cups (60 g) fresh lemon verbena or 2 cups (112 g) dried lemon verbena

1 cup (30 g) fresh rose petals or 1 cup (96 g) dried rose petals

1 cup (96 g) fresh orange peel pieces or 1 cup (64 g) dried orange peel pieces

¼ cup (24 g) celery seed

## SLEEPY TIME BATH

*This is a calming synthesis of herbs that will assist you in releasing the day. Wash your worries down the drain and tuck yourself in for a night of deep and peaceful sleep.*

8 quarts (8 L) water

½ cup (180 g) fresh oatstraw or ½ cup (24 g) dried oatstraw

½ cup (36 g) fresh lavender or ½ cup (8 g) dried lavender

½ cup (36 g) fresh whole chamomile or ½ cup (8 g) dried whole chamomile

## SORE JOINTS BATH

4 gallons (16 L) water

½ cup (96 g) fresh juniper berries or ½ cup (40 g) dried juniper berries

½ cup (15 g) fresh basil leaves or ½ cup (24 g) dried basil leaves

½ cup (48 g) fresh orange peel pieces or ½ cup (32 g) dried orange peel pieces

¼ cup (12 g) fresh rosemary or ¼ cup (13 g) dried rosemary leaves

¼ cup (24 g) celery seed

## SUMMERTIME COOLING BATH

*Make a tea with peppermint, let it cool down, and pour it into your bath. Add freshly sliced lemons to the bathwater and cool off.*

8 quarts (8 L) water

1 cup (48 g) fresh peppermint leaves or 1 cup (96 g) dried peppermint leaves

2 lemons, sliced

## SWEET DREAMS FOOT BATH

*This is quite relaxing and a great end-of-the-day treatment.*

4 quarts (4 L) water

½ cup (36 g) fresh lavender or ½ cup (8 g) dried lavender

½ cup (15 g) fresh rose petals or ½ cup (48 g) dried rose petals

1 teaspoon (2 g) powdered nutmeg

## TENSION TAMER FOOT BATH

4 quarts (4 L) water

1 cup (72 g) fresh lavender flower or 1 cup (16 g) dried lavender

½ cup (90 g) fresh oatstraw or ½ cup (24 g) dried oatstraw

½ cup (48 g) fresh lemon balm or ½ cup (48 g) dried lemon balm

# Glossary

**adaptogen:** Enhances ability to deal with emotional, physical, and environmental stress.

**alterative:** Aids the body in elimination processes. Alters the body's condition, helping to normalize and restore healthy body function.

**analgesic:** Produces a pain-relieving effect.

**anesthetic:** Causes temporary loss of body sensation, used in pain-relief protocols.

**anthelmintic:** Inhibits and expels parasites.

**antibacterial:** Kills bacteria directly or inhibits bacterial growth.

**anticatarrhal:** Reduces inflammation of the mucous membrane, reduces excess mucus.

**antifungal:** Kills fungus directly or inhibits fungal growth.

**anti-inflammatory:** Decreases inflammation and counteracts the effects of inflammation.

**antioxidant:** Limits and prevents oxidation and tissue damage.

**antispasmodic:** Relieves cramps and spasms.

**antiviral:** Fights viral infections.

**aperient:** Has a gentle laxative action.

**astringent:** Tightens and contracts tissue, decreasing excess moisture and secretions.

**bitter tonic:** Bitter-tasting herbs that stimulate digestion.

**carminative:** Increases digestive capacity, promotes peristalsis, dispels gas, and relieves gas pain.

**cholagogue:** Promotes the flow of bile.

**circulatory stimulant:** Increases the flow of blood to tissue.

**demulcent:** Decreases inflammation and soothes and protects the mucous membrane.

**diuretic:** Increases urination.

**emmenagogue:** Promotes menstruation.

**emollient:** Softens and protects the skin.

**expectorant:** Expels excess mucus from the respiratory system.

**galactagogue:** Increases the flow and quality of breast milk.

**hemostat:** Stops the flow of blood.

**nervine:** Soothes, calms, relaxes, and strengthens the nervous system.

**nutritive:** Contains vitamins and minerals that nourish the body.

**rubefacient:** Stimulates circulation in the skin.

**tonic:** Increases overall wellness.

**vulnerary:** Soothes and heals inflamed and injured tissue.

# Sources

## HERBAL EDUCATION

Living Awareness Institute
*www.livingawareness.com*

Blue Otter School of Herbal Medicine
*www.blueotterschool.com*

California School of Herbal Studies
*www.cshs.com*

Dandelion Herbal Center
*www.dandelionherb.com*

Dhyana Center of Health Sciences
*www.dhyanacenter.com*

EverGreen Herb School of Integrative Herbology
*www.evergreenherbgarden.org*

Rosalee de la Forêt
*www.herbswithrosalee.com*

Sage Mountain Herbal Retreat Center & Botanical Sanctuary
*www.sagemountain.com*

Southwest School of Botanical Medicine
*www.swsbm.com*

The Bellebuono School of Herbal Medicine
*www.hollybellebuono.com*

United Plant Savers
*www.unitedplantsavers.org*

## DRIED HERBS

*Mountain Rose Herbs*
*www.mountainroseherbs.com*
What herb do you want? They have it!

Pacific Botanicals
*www.pacificbotanicals.com*
I have been buying herbs from Pacific Botanicals since I first started working with herbs. The herbs are always in excellent condition, and I have never been disappointed.

## GHEE

Pure Indian Foods
*www.pureindianfoods.com*
Pure Indian Foods make excellent ghee. Their butter comes from grass-fed cows.

## NURSERIES

Crimson Sage Medicinal Plants Nursery
*www.crimson-sage.com*

Horizon Herbs
*www.strictlymedicinalseeds.com*
Horizon Herbs has an extensive selection
of medicinal and culinary seeds and
herb plants that can be shipped to your
doorstep.

Morningsun Herb Farm
*www.morningsunherbfarm.com*
Morningsun Herb Farm carries a huge
variety of medicinal and culinary herbs
and can ship them anywhere in the
country.

## SEEDS

Baker Creek Heirloom Seeds
*www.rareseeds.com*

Seed Savers Exchange
*www.seedsaversexchange.org*

Territorial Seed Company
*www.territorialseed.com*
They offer a wonderful variety of organic
herb and vegetable seeds.

## BOTTLES AND JARS

ebottles.com
*www.ebottles.com*
They carry a wide variety of all kinds of
bottles and jars at reasonable prices. There
is a $50 purchasing minimum.

Specialty Bottle
*www.specialtybottle.com*
Specialty Bottle carries any plastic, glass,
or metal bottle or jar you could ever
imagine.

Sunburst Bottle Company
*www.sunburstbottle.com*
I have ordered bottles and jars here for
almost twenty years. They cater to home
crafters and have a wide selection.

# Bibliography

Bergner, Paul. *The Healing Power of Minerals, Special Nutrients, and Trace Elements.* Rocklin, CA: Prima Press, 1997

Dawson, Adele. *Health, Happiness and the Pursuit of Herbs.* Lexington, MA: The Stephen Greene Press, 1980.

Duke, James A. *The Green Pharmacy.* Emmaus, PA: Rodale Press, 1997.

Fallon, Sally. *Nourishing Traditions: The Cookbook that Challenges Politically Correct Nutrition and the Diet Dictocrats.* 2nd ed. Washington, DC: New Trends Publishing, 1999.

Flaws, Bob. *The Tao of Healthy Eating: Dietary Wisdom According to Traditional Chinese Medicine.* Boulder, CO: Blue Poppy Press, 1998.

Frawley, David, and Vasant Lad. *The Yoga of Herbs: An Ayurvedic Guide to Herbal Medicine.* Twin Lakes, WI: Lotus Press, 1992.

Gladstar, Rosemary. *Rosemary Gladstar's Herbal Recipes for Vibrant Health.* North Adams, MA: Storey Books, 2001.

Hemphill, Ian, and Elizabeth Hemphill. *Sticks, Seeds, Pods & Leaves: A Cook's Guide to Culinary Spices and Herbs.* Victoria, Australia: Hardie Grant Books, 2007.

Holmes, Peter. *The Energetics of Western Herbs.* 3rd ed. Boulder, CO: Snow Lotus Press, 1997.

Le, Kim. *The Simple Path to Health: A Guide to Oriental Nutrition and Well-Being.* 2nd ed. Portland, OR: Rudra Press, 1996.

Mills, Simon, and Kerry Bone. *Principles and Practice of Phytotherapy: Modern Herbal Medicine.* St. Louis, MO: Churchill Livingstone, 2000.

Mitchell, William A. *Plant Medicine in Practice: Using the Teachings of John Bastyr.* St Louis, MO: Churchill Livingstone, 2003.

Moore, Michael. *Medicinal Plants of the Mountain West.* 2nd ed. Santa Fe, NM: Museum of New Mexico Press, 2003.

Moore, Michael. *Medicinal Plants of the Pacific West.* Santa Fe, NM: Red Crane Books, 1993.

Packard, Candis C. *Pocket Guide to Ayurvedic Healing.* Freedon, CA: The Crossing Press, 1996.

Pedersen, Mark. *Nutritional Herbology: A Reference Guide to Herbs.* 4th ed. Warsaw, IN: Wendell W. Whitman Company, 1998.

Pitchford, Paul. *Healing with Whole Foods: Asian Traditions and Modern Nutrition.* 2nd ed. Berkeley, CA: North Atlantic Books, 1996.

Pole, Sebastian. *Ayurvedic Medicine: The Principles of Traditional Practice.* St. Louis, MO: Churchill Livingstone, 2006.

Price, Weston A. *Nutrition and Physical Degeneration.* 14th ed. La Mesa, CA: Price-Pottenger Nutrition Foundation, 2000.

Schmid, Ronald F. *Traditional Foods are Your Best Medicine: Improving Health and Nutrition with Native Nutrition.* 3rd ed. Rochester, VT: Healing Arts Press, 1997.

Tierra, Michael. *The Way of Herbs.* 2nd ed. New York, NY: Washington Square Press, 1983.

Willard, Terry. *Textbook of Modern Herbology.* 2nd ed. Alberta, Canada: Wild Rose College of Natural Healing, 1993.

# Index

# About the Author

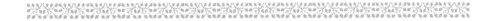

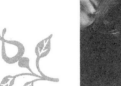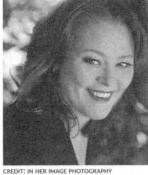

CREDIT: IN HER IMAGE PHOTOGRAPHY

**Kami McBride** has taught herbal medicine for more than thirty years and has helped thousands of people learn to use herbs as the centerpiece of their proactive health care plan. She has taught herbal medicine at the University of California School of Nursing and the California Institute of Integral Studies and leads workshops and online courses that help people bring the healing power of herbs into their daily lives to create self-reliance and revitalize their relationship with the plant world. Visit Kami at *www.kamimcbride.com*.

# From the Author

Thanks for grabbing a copy of *The Herbal Kitchen*! I poured my heart into this book and I know you are going to enjoy it. To show my appreciation, I have a special gift for you—The Turmeric Sessions—a video series where I show you how to make my favorite recipes using turmeric, a powerful anti-inflammatory and antioxidant. You can get access to this free digital gift full of turmeric goodness here: *www.turmericsessions.com/freegift.*

# Ready to bring *The Herbal Kitchen* to life?

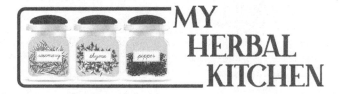

If you're excited to bring herbs into the heart of your home, you can join Kami in the MY HERBAL KITCHEN video course where she'll guide you step by step in how to create herbal pantry favorites.

Some people go for it and dig right into the 250 recipes in *The Herbal Kitchen* book and others really enjoy having this online video tutorial course to support them along the way. Kami will walk you through core herbal recipes and everything you need to know to set up your own herbal kitchen so you can put the flavor enhancing and health benefits of culinary herbs to work right away.

You can get started at www.myherbalkitchen.com

# To Our Readers

Conari Press, an imprint of Red Wheel/Weiser, publishes books on topics ranging from spirituality, personal growth, and relationships to women's issues, parenting, and social issues. Our mission is to publish quality books that will make a difference in people's lives—how we feel about ourselves and how we relate to one another. We value integrity, compassion, and receptivity, both in the books we publish and in the way we do business.

Our readers are our most important resources, and we value your input, suggestions, and ideas about what you would like to see published. Please feel free to contact us, to request our latest book catalog, or to be added to our mailing list.

**CONARI PRESS**
An imprint of Red Wheel/Weiser, LLC
65 Parker Street, Suite 7
Newburyport, MA 01950
*www.redwheelweiser.com*